Katrin
Girls *Do* Do That

*The Yoga Sutra Teachings
On Healing Yourself,
And How They Reached Tibet*

By Geshe Michael Roach

Published in 2022 by

Diamond Cutter Press
6490 State Route 179
Sedona, Arizona 86351
USA

www.diamondcutterpress.com

Book design by Rosa van Grieken and Gina Rivera

ISBN 978-1-937114-32-9
ISBN 978-1-937114-31-2 (eBook)

Printed in the United States of America

Part One
Girls *Do* Do That

The old man stared down at the bowl of tea in his hands for another long moment, and then set the steel eyes on me again, studying my face intently.

And then finally he said, "The thing you ask... the thing you ask to learn, it is a very serious thing." He paused again, and his eyes fell silently, as if seeking words beneath the surface of the tea.

"And even if I knew—a little—about this... healing... well I could never teach it to you." A sharp flash of pain burst through my chest. He saw it.

"I mean, without knowing... without knowing exactly who you are, and why you want to learn this thing; why you, why someone so young, why just a girl."

He paused once more, studying his bowl, turning it in his fingers. And then suddenly he looked up again, his eyes flashing.

"And how you found me! How you found this hermitage! I don't believe anyone has ever reached this place the way you did!"

He leaned over into my eyes and my life again and he said, "So now tell me child, from the beginning, and leave nothing out."

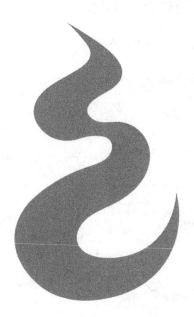

Table of Contents

1.

Our Home

I was born in the Water Pig year of the First Cycle, or 1083 by Western counting. My very first memory is opening my eyes, and looking up, and seeing an exquisite dark-blue turquoise dangling in the air above me, jiggling and dancing happily. It was framed in small rings of silver with a color like moonlight, and the rings hung from a string of beautiful walnut-colored wooden beads.

My eyes followed the beads up to strong, lovely brown fingers, and then over them I caught my first sight of my beloved brother Tenzing, his handsome high-cheeked face framed in the steel blue of the round sky-window, far above. His bright brown doe eyes sparkled down at me with love, and he laughed aloud, and cried out, "Amala! My pretty baby sister has finally woken up!"

Amala, which means, "my dear Mother" in our language, came and leaned over, and I looked up and saw her dear face in the sky too. She hugged my brother Tenzing, and gave his smooth-shaven head an affectionate rub, and said, "Oh yes, she is so pretty. But now you come and get back to your studies, my little Geshe, and let the girl have her rest."

He smiled with that irresistible snow-white smile of his, and said goodbye gently with his happy eyes. The two faces disappeared from the circle of sky, and the precious turquoise was pulled gently away, and I was left in my cradle of soft woolens and warm yak-hair blankets, still looking up at the blue of the new day.

I remember laying there for hours, gazing up through the sky-window of our tent-house. The lovely yellow Sun would cross the round window slowly as the day passed, throwing a shaft of gold down to me, a pillar of light in which spirals and wisps of smoke from the family fire would play for me all day long. The warm round patch of light at the bottom would cross the room and my body lazily, warm from above, and below my back the warmth of the family fire spread from a stone-lined pit beneath the sky-window.

I lived in the window; it was all I could see, and I felt like a sister to the Sun at day, and the

Moon at night, when it crossed the circle of darkness on the same path the Sun had taken earlier. My heart would leave from the window then, and circle above as the bright white fire of the stars did, around some mighty unseen axis. I was a baby in the Sky, and rarely thought of Earth.

The sky-window was the best part of our tent-house, or yurt. It was a great open circle of sturdy juniper wood, about four feet across—it bathed the whole house in a soft amber light, and let the fireplace smoke out to the sky. Eight arching spokes crossed it, broken by a smaller circle of wood about a foot across—and inside this circle there was a lovely wooden cross.

The round window frame was itself held high by several dozen roof poles—these were painted a russet orange, with intricate smaller designs like dragons and firebirds in indigo, crimson, and an emerald green. Looking up from my cradle, lost in the pillar of sunlight and the spokes that radiated out from it, I sometimes felt as though I was within my own body, within the very core that ran up and down it, gazing at the lines of radiant vessels spreading out from the core. And so these are my first memories, of a great axis and lines of light, with the spheres of stars and planets transversing them, within and all around me—my new home.

Our home was a warm and lively one. Like all families where I lived, we all slept together, spreading woolen carpets and blankets and quilts all across the floor in the evening, talking and laughing and singing as we settled down. On one side of the yurt my grandmother, whose name was Tara, had a special straw mattress and some fine covered chests, so she was a little higher and would sit in the firelight, peaceful and strong, gazing down at us with her laughing, sparkling eyes, looking like a queen. And indeed she had been a queen, or a princess, of her people in the very far north, near a great lake named Baikal.

"Tell me the story again, Grandmother Tara," I would beg as I sat in her lap as a girl. She would set aside the spindle she was using to make yarn for my mother Amala's carpets, and gladly, for she really was a princess at heart and never did enjoy hand work. Then as expected her hands would go to the pouch at her bright sash belt, and pull out a piece of *chura kampo* for me. This was our candy as children in those days, for sugar cane could never grow so high, and the "white sand" (as we called sugar) had to be carried over the mountains from India on beasts of burden—so it was rare and precious.

Chura kampo was even better though, small cubes of cheese a little larger than dice for a game, strung on a string and dried in the sun. Our land was so high that almost nothing ever spoiled, and the little squares would last for years. They were as hard as rocks; you had to suck on them for hours, which was a good way to keep children quiet during a story. (Uncle claimed that the dried cheese squares were the invention of evil spirits, because everyone in Tibet ate them, and couldn't say their prayers for hours at a time when their mouths were jammed full.) But Grandmother Tara never said hello or goodbye to me without pulling out a piece and tucking it into my mouth.

2.

The Family

"I was young and beautiful then," Grandmother would begin, and it was easy to believe, because even in her old age she cut a striking figure. Her waist-length hair had long since gone pure white, but it was still full and shining—she would plait it into a single braid, like most of the Tibetan women, but then take it around her head and tie it up in the back with ribbons of Bengal silk, looking always as though she wore a crown.

Her blouses too were silk, with long sleeves that came well down past her fingers, an old custom of nobility to show that they never did menial tasks—and not bad for wrapping your hands on a cold day either. She would always sew the blouses with a high Chinese collar that complimented her long neck and aristocratic chin, which she carried high—not out of vanity, but from the natural bearing of royalty that never left her. It was from her too that my brother Tenzing had gotten his high sculpted cheeks, and elegant aquiline nose.

"My father was a high chieftain in our land, and a renowned merchant. He led a great caravan south and westward to the Silk Road, seeking to trade musk and furs and precious metals from our forests. I had pestered him to take me along, just once, and he finally agreed—although I think it was mostly from fear of losing me to bands of raiders from the eastern Mongol lands, which even then were gathering strength.

"Near the ancient city of Khotan, we ran into another caravan on the Silk Road itself, this one headed to China proper with woolen goods and hordes of sheep. It was led by your dear Grandfather..." and she would always pause to wipe a tear from her eye, for he had passed away before I was born "...who was as you know one of the greatest traders Tibet has ever known; not that he was so rich in those days, that was before he met me. And of course you know it was he who taught your father everything he knows, back when he was just a young fellow with a few bags of salt and a couple of yaks," and she smiled indulgently (I did tell you, I think, that she was from my mother's side of the family).

"So to make a long story short, your grandfather laid eyes on me once and was so smitten that he ordered the caravan stopped, and spent three weeks practically on his hands and knees begging my father for my hand, while the camel and yak drivers from both camps traded *chang* beer and *arak* wine and drank and fought until nearly all the goods were ruined. In the end Grandfather parted with half his entire wealth—300 sheep—and I rode away with him," she would finish proudly, and I would have a vision of a vast sea of fluffy sheep headed west, while Grandfather and his prize rode two single horses east. In later times, I came to realize that my grandfather had made a shrewd alliance with the Mongols, who were to build one of the greatest empires Asia has ever seen; the marriage protected our family and its caravans for many years.

But for me Grandmother Tara was like another little girl, and we would sit and giggle together for hours, much to my mother Amala's consternation, since she needed yarn for her carpets. Grandmother taught me to make the morning offering of sang—dried powder of juniper boughs from the heights of sacred mountains—to the Tengeri, the sky gods of the Mongols. When she kneeled over the smoke rising from the fire pit, she looked like a Priestess Queen, and I was in awe of her power and grace. In my world she was the firmament, unshakable authority and strength.

Father, like the true businessman he was, would put up with all this hocus-pocus good-naturedly. He was of course a devout follower of the Buddha, but would go on special trips to make sure his mother-in-law always had her sacred juniper powder, "Because you have to cover yourself, you know? Who knows which religion might end up being right!"

This kind of tolerance was the basis of his philosophy of life, and although he was often gone on caravans I loved and respected him deeply. He was a ferocious bargainer, so persuasive that my brother Tenzing and I would always avoid him in the morning, when it was time for chores to be handed out, because within a few minutes he would have talked you into doing extra jobs and still feeling that you were letting the family down somehow. He was brilliant in business the way his brother, Uncle Jampa, was in spiritual things. And in fact at the heart of Father's business he always lived by a single rule—that both sides in a business deal must profit from the deal. In this he embodied in real life the most important code we were brought up on: to take care of others as well as we would take care of ourselves.

Father's main business was in salt and the fine woolen carpets that Amala and other women would weave in their yurts. He and the menfolk from several other families would lead a long line of yaks and other pack animals northeast to the great salt flats, and then down south to the passes overlooking Nepal. They would ride into that great valley and trade in the bustling capital of Kathmandu, mostly for precious items from India, still further to the south. He'd come home with sugar and rice; saffron and sandalwood and other spices and scents; and the treasured silks of Varanasi, on the banks of the great Ganges River.

Father's people even had some Indian blood, and he sported a happy chubby face with round eyes and a foreigner's nose, which made it easy for him to trade even in the outlying lands. In fact he had even travelled—along with his brother and sister—with my other grandfather as far as central India, in the early days.

Father was the baby of the three, and Uncle Jampa, who lived with us, was in the middle. The sister was much older, but she was gone, and no one ever spoke about her.

My mother, Amala, was a quiet, nervous woman. Her face must have taken after Grandfather's, for it was nothing like Grandmother's, but rather thin and pointed, with wide-open owl's eyes and jet black hair. Her life was hard with my father gone so much, and she took every responsibility upon herself. With the exception of a milkmaid named Bukla and a few field workers at planting and harvest, Amala refused the help freely offered by the families of my father's caravan mates, whose wives and children camped nearby to the east whenever the men were on the road. And so we rarely had visitors.

Amala would spend the whole day with her carpets, weaving on a loom across the fire pit from Grandmother's little throne. The loom was pushed up against the wall of the yurt, which was made of a wooden lattice higher than a man where it met the roof poles. If Father came home with a special order for a large carpet for some Nepalese estate or temple, Amala would set up a wider loom on a beam that went from the top of the wall to one of the two stout juniper trunks set on either side of the fire pit as supports for the sky-window and the roof.

Amala's carpets were famous for their intricate designs, more detailed than those of any other weaver in our part of the country. She was a master not only of the Tibetan snow-lions and mountain scenes but also of the complex symbols from China; the art of the wax-seals of the Mongol princes; and the forms of the fearsome jungle animals of India. For hours while I sat distracting

20

my Grandmother on one side of the family fire, Amala would labor with resignation at the loom across from us, combining these different worlds within the new world of the wooden frame. She slapped down every new line of yarn with a heavy wooden bar, in a rhythm that sank into me and stayed, along with the secrets of the designs, for I was a curious girl—I watched carefully and learned them all.

The only thing that could break Amala away from her daylong trance at the loom was the entrance of my brother Tenzing every hour or two, coming to get more Tibetan tea for Uncle as he taught the classes in his yurt across the clearing from ours. This tea is a staple in our country, and more like a broth. We would drink 15 or 20 cups a day to give energy at our high altitude, and to protect us from the cold. Every morning and afternoon, Amala would prepare a new batch, filling the huge tea churn with boiling water, chunks of pressed japak tea leaves from China, milk, butter, salt, and often baking soda or nutmeg. Then she would seal the lid of the churn, which was a long thin barrel that looked like a cannon set on end, beautiful worn hardwood with ornate brass rings. After that came the familiar whoosh of the plunger, forced down through the tea over and over until it was a thick golden soup which, for us, was the real sign of Home.

Tenzing would bring in Uncle's smaller churn and fill it, while Amala fussed over "my little Geshe" and asked him how classes were going. One of the first things I remember ever saying to my mother was, "Amala, I want to go hear Uncle's classes too. "

She peered down at me with a look of faint surprise and said, "But girls don't do that, dear."

Suddenly I heard a voice in my head, very loud, and it said "Girls *do* do that!" But like a good girl in an eleventh-century Asian family I didn't make a peep, just looked down at my feet.

And so the only time I really had my brother Tenzing to myself, away from Uncle and Amala, was at night when we lay down on Amala's lush carpets with our heads to the family fire, nestled safely between Grandmother's bed on one side and my father and mother atop a higher stack of carpets on the other. We would pull the covers over our heads and wait for the sound of the adults all sleeping, and then I would ask Tenzing what Uncle had taught them that day.

He would lecture me proudly, as if he were already a Geshe, and answer all my questions with love and patience. Then one night he burst out, "Friday, today I found out something really special!"

"What's that?" I whispered back.

"Uncle has a secret!" he announced.

3.

How I Got My Name

"So tell me!" I whispered, louder.

"One of the other boys, you know, the big one, Drom, he sneaked a little toad into class. And he was pushing it around between him and his friend Hammer and Hammer tried to pick it up without Uncle seeing what was going on and..." Tenzing started to giggle like crazy.

Whenever he giggled I had to giggle, but I managed a loud "Shhh! You'll wake everybody up! So what happened?"

"So the toad, you know like they do, he pee-peed right in Hammer's hand, and he yelped, and tossed the toad over towards Uncle's altar."

"Then what happened?"

"Uncle was busy looking up some quotation that he couldn't remember, and didn't even notice. I figured everybody would get in trouble if we didn't get the toad back before Uncle saw it, so I pretended to get up to fill Uncle's tea cup again."

"How'd you get the toad?"

"On the way past the altar I acted like I dropped the top to the churn and it rolled off towards the back of the altar, and I stooped down and squeezed myself between the wall of the yurt and the altar and reached way back for the toad, and then I felt that one of the stones in the back of the altar was loose, and I peeked in and saw that you could slide it out, and it looked like there was a little package inside there."

"Did you see what was in it?"

"Oh no! Just then Uncle said 'Aha! There you are!' and I thought he was talking to me and I grabbed the toad in one hand and the wood lid in the other and held up the lid and said 'Got it!' and saw Uncle still had his head down and was reading some line to the class. So I went up and filled his cup and I was shaking and almost put the toad on the churn instead of the lid, and you know Drom— he was already smirking at me, so I sat back down and on the way I dropped the toad in his lap. It was great."

"So what do you think is in the secret package?" I asked urgently.

"I don't know, and I don't see how we'll ever find out. Uncle almost never leaves his yurt for more than a few minutes—just to pet the cows or go to the toilet."

I nodded knowingly, for Uncle was indeed single-minded. He was a monk's monk, and stuck to his prayers and studies late into the night. He was on sort of a permanent loan to our family from the local monastery, to do what we call *shapten*. Father had acquired, from a temple in Kathmandu, a complete set of the ancient teachings of the Buddha that had been translated so far into our tongue from Sanskrit, the very old sacred language of India. This was before printing from woodblocks was very common in our country, and the books were hand-copied onto long thin sheaves of rice paper, modelled after the ancient leaves of palm fronds that had been the first paper of India. The copyists had illuminated each page with paintings of angels and wise ones, in dyes made from crushing precious stones.

These books were nearly priceless and were our family's greatest treasure. *Shapten* was a custom where a monk-scholar would be sent from the local monastery to stay for a while with a family that possessed even a single precious book. The monk would sing the book out loud, slowly, while the members of the family wandered in and out of the room, listening often without understanding, hoping to plant a blessing to learn the contents of the book properly in a future lifetime.

And so Uncle's job was to chant our manuscripts out loud, and I cannot recall a time in the early years of my life when he was not going through them once more, singing as often as not only to the cows and stars, long into the night. He was getting on in years, and it was common late in the evening to peek in his little wood door, before the rest of the family went to sleep, and see him stooped over with his forehead pressed against the breast of some exquisite angel on a page, fallen fast asleep in the middle of a sentence.

A monk like Uncle who came to sing the holy books for a family would be given a separate place to stay, since by his vows he could not sleep where there was a woman under the same roof. If the match between the visiting monk and the family worked out well, though, he might stay on for a longer and longer time, becoming a friend and teacher and sort of counselor to the whole family; and each member would feel free to drop in almost any time to get his advice on both matters of the spirit and business of the day. And this, as

Grandmother Tara told me the story, is how I came to get my name.

Several days after I was born, Father and Amala wrapped me up and walked over to Uncle's yurt, for it is a custom in our land for a Lama to give the child his or her name. Grandmother came along to make sure everything was done just right, according to tradition.

After the formalities—ritual greetings and bows, small offerings of animal hide filled with butter, and blocks of fine black tea—we settled down on a rug before Uncle, who like most monks used his small wooden bed as the only chair in his small home.

With a nervous glance at Grandmother, Father began: "Esteemed Lama, venerable one, Jampa Rabgay La, we ask that you do us the honor of granting our daughter a name."

Uncle beamed in his usual way, a wide white smile under a few long straggly white wisps of mustache, drooping over the corners of his mouth. But his eyes were still sad, with some deep sadness that he held as long as I ever knew him. "Certainly! Certainly! With pleasure!" he rasped.

Uncle gazed at each of us warmly, pausing at Grandmother's stern eyes, and continued, "Now it's going to take time though. Things have to be done right, you know. There's a few steps I have to be going through to get just the right name, so everyone bear with me. Especially you, little girl!" and he reached down and tickled me under the chin. I frowned a bit—to be different—but spared him a crying spell, because I really did feel very happy in the bright warmth of his yurt and his presence.

Then with another glance at Grandmother, who was sitting up stern and tall behind Father and Amala, Uncle fumbled around in some covered baskets he kept stacked near his bed. Finally he pulled out a small lacquered box with two small white bones in it. These were the knuckles of a sheep, almost square, and had different indentations on each side. This made them very popular among the Mongols and Northern Tribes as dice, for playing games or for telling the future. Grandmother had grown up with these, and nodded her approval.

Then Uncle took down a small book of loose leaves of rice paper wrapped in a grimy old silken cloth, worn with generations of use. It was a book of *kartsi*, about the positions of the stars and planets, full of strange drawings and symbols for helping to determine the best days to do important jobs, and which days to avoid, and hints for making all kinds of decisions. Uncle used to tell me later that kindness and an understanding of how good deeds really worked were actually the only two things that anyone needed to make any decision, but that both of these considerations also demanded that we respect the customs which others might feel were important. And so he leafed through the book carefully, humming significantly from time to time, throwing the dice on the little table between him and my parents, calculating on the joints of his fingers the way we Tibetans do, and making occasional notes on a little scrap of parchment with a bamboo stylus, in his beautiful, deliberate style of calligraphy.

He went on quite long, and despite themselves all the adults began to get a little restless. Thankfully I was enjoying the feeling of the moment, still quiet. He frowned. He mumbled to himself. He glanced nervously at Grandmother from time to time, and she began to feel some concern. Finally Uncle gave a long sigh; stacked the pages of the book back together and folded the cloth over them; and then placed the dice back in their box. He did all this very slowly, as if to delay a difficult moment. Even my parents were beginning to feel nervous, and Grandmother was close to alarmed.

"The girl's name," uttered Uncle slowly, looking from one face to another, "must be... Pasang."

Grandmother jolted, and then glared at Uncle. "Is there some danger?" she asked. "Should the girl be kept in a kettle?"

Uncle shook his head nervously, for Grandmother could be difficult when the world deviated from her plan for it. He had travelled widely, and knew of the Northern custom of keeping a newborn child in a large kettle for several days, if the mother had lost children in birthing before. People thought that death spirits would be out and about looking for the newest child, and so the babe would be hidden, and everyone would speak about it as if it were already dead. This they said would fool the spirits, and they would go away. The mother would nurse her baby at quiet moments in a darkened tent or yurt, under a cloth.

"No," said Uncle thoughtfully, and then he added his favorite phrase: "Things are not always what they seem." He paused a moment, and continued. "No need to fool the spirits; quite the contrary, in fact."

"Then why have you given her a boy's name, if not to confuse death spirits who are seeking her?" demanded Grandmother, for she felt that my mother must know the truth, even if it was hard.

And here Amala herself spoke quietly, more trusting of the Lama, and more resigned to his decisions. "It is a good name," she began, "and I have known many fine people with the same name. Do you give it to her because she was born on Friday?" For this too is commonplace in our land, to name children from the day of the week on which they were born—and Pasang is our word for Friday.

"No," replied Uncle carefully, "no, not even that. And please," he held up his hand gently, "please, it is not I who have chosen her name," he looked at Grandmother. "It *is* her name; it *must* be her name. Everything is in agreement," he said with a note of finality, waving at the ancient book and the box of dice.

"But what does it mean, my brother?" spoke Father finally, in the quiet, thoughtful way he had sometimes, when his mind went higher, beyond the grand sweep of his business ventures.

Uncle turned his sad face and joined his beautiful eyes to my father's own. He spoke softly, almost reverently. "Her name is Pasang, and you shall call her this; she will be called Friday. But remember always that the real meaning of the word *pasang* is the planet Venus, the morning star. The star rises, far brighter than any other star in the entire night, in the entire sky, to signal the end of darkness, and the coming of the Sun. Pasang, Friday, Venus—the morning star..." he said quietly, and touched his warm soft hands to my head. "She comes in the darkest and coldest hour of the night, she knows the worst of times, and then the radiance rises from the East, and swallows her in glory, a glory that fills the world." There was a silence then, and a feeling of something to be, and it satisfied even Grandmother Tara.

4.

I Start on a Different Path

Uncle Jampa though was rightly valued in the village of Kishong and the nearby monastery of Gempil Ling not for his powers of divination, but for his knowledge of the ancient books and the wisdom passed down through the many generations of kind and thoughtful teachers, first in the land of India and then our own Tibet. Uncle was unique in that he could read the old books in the Mother Tongue, in Sanskrit, and he had trained in India for some twelve years with one of the greatest sages of our time.

His knowledge and humility and good humor made Uncle a popular teacher, and for most of the late morning and afternoon he would conduct classes for groups of young student monks who made the long walk from the monastery each day to bask in his knowledge and get outside the abbey walls for a few hours' fun, strolling through the countryside without any supervision.

Classes lasted about an hour each, beginning with the junior students first, and then working up to the more experienced ones by evening. In our day there were around 250 monks at Gempil Ling; about ten of these were senior teachers, like Uncle, who had responsibility for instructing the student monks—these numbered about 120. The student monks were divided into ten classes, according to their level in the ten-year course leading to the title of Geshe. A Geshe was a monk who had mastered the five great ancient books on subjects ranging from philosophy to prayer and meditation. The course was quite difficult, and only a few monks in each class passed the final examinations. Ours was one of the first monasteries in Tibet to train monks this way, and Uncle—with the training he had gained in India—had helped organize the curriculum of study and methods of examinations.

Over the course of many years, the training and title of the Geshe later became even more elaborate and rigorous, and spread throughout our country. But even in our time, it was every monk's hope at Gempil Ling to attain this honor, and every mother's dream to see her son stand for the oral examinations and win the peaked golden hat, before a crowd of villagers and monks. Certainly it was my mother's lifetime dream for my brother Tenzing.

Tenzing was almost ten years older than me, and before I was even born had been dedicated by my parents to the monk's life. Boys as young as seven were allowed to take their first vows—the ancient tradition was that they only had to be big enough to yell at a wild crow and scare it from its perch. These novices spent their first eight years learning to read, and sometimes to write; they also devoted several hours a day to committing at least three of the ancient classics to memory. Only when they reached the age of fifteen—when they were deemed old enough to reason out a question carefully—did they begin formal studies with a teacher to learn the meaning of the books they had already memorized.

From then on it was ten years of hard study—which nowadays has stretched into twenty—to reach the Geshe exams. Halfway through, at age twenty, the young man made his final choice about whether to remain a monk or not. This time the decision was his own, and it must be kept for life. But girls had no such choice, as I learned the hard way.

My father and uncle had wheedled the abbot of the monastery, an old friend of theirs who had also done some study in India, to allow Tenzing to become Uncle's attendant. This was all instigated by Amala, who wanted to have her cake and eat it too: she wanted her dear son to be a Geshe, but also to be close to us as he grew up. Young attendants of a senior Lama would do things like fetching their meals from the kitchen; hauling water for drinking and washing from a nearby stream, in two buckets hanging from a pole balanced across their shoulders; and keeping the Lama's altar clean, with fresh flowers and offerings of scented water for the angels. But the most important job of all was keeping the Lama's cup filled with hot, strong, salty Tibetan tea—which, as everyone knows, is absolutely essential for thinking clearly while you read a difficult book.

One day Tenzing was late coming to get the tea; Amala was distracted repairing a crooked section of rug, and Grandmother had decided to take a nap. I was about five years old—I remember. I just boldly got up and did something I'd always wanted to do. I snatched up a small churn of tea and took it to Uncle.

As I slipped into his door, Uncle was in mid-sentence, looking down intently from his seat on his bed at a group of eight young beginners, Tenzing's own class.

"... And so the real protection—the real shelter and refuge—is not the pictures of holy beings, or even the books they taught in our world," he said intensely, waving to the altar and the stack of precious manuscripts. "Rather, it is the ideas themselves that protect you: doing good to others and knowing why you do, and knowing what it will bring..." Suddenly he stopped, and stared over the little huddle of shaven heads, and caught me with a surprised look.

I glanced down quickly and, before his eyes could tell me otherwise, marched up to the front of the room, along a little space in front of the altar left by the students for the attendant to pass. I reached Uncle's table and stood off to the side. Suddenly the silence struck me, and I felt the pressure of the boys' eyes on me. My hands began to shake. I took off the lid of the small wooden churn and lifted it up to fill Uncle's cup, but I wasn't tall enough. One of the boys started to titter.

I remember, it is all very clear to me, because it determined the different path I took in life I think, just those few moments. I set the churn down on the floor and reached out with both hands to grasp the cup. Somebody muttered, "A girl... in the class!" I didn't look to see who it was, and it didn't matter. I heard what I heard.

My hands now were shaking so badly I had to tuck the churn under my arm, and use both hands to hold the cup. The tea started to come out.

And then Uncle said, "Friday... Friday! What are you doing?"

I started and sloshed some of the tea on the floor. Several boys began to giggle and snicker. There was only a little tea in the cup but I couldn't go on. I looked up at Uncle helplessly.

"I... I... brought your... t-t-tea," I stammered, with the churn under my arm. I couldn't reach high enough to get the cup back up on the table. So I just held it out towards Uncle, and he rescued me then; with his warm hands on mine, he took the cup, and laid his soft sad eyes on mine, searchingly, but with comfort.

"Thank you Friday," he said, kindly, but in the way of dismissing me from the room. I stepped backwards away from him, as attendants do, but a very loud, indignant little voice went off inside my head. "Stay!" it said. "Stand there!" it said. "He is going to tell them the rest about protection, and it is important for everyone, and you have a right to know about it too!"

As it did then, this voice has come to me throughout my life. Sometimes I think it's just pride, or some other negative emotion. But oftentimes it orders me to do something for the sake of truth itself. And either way, it is always telling me to do something which is difficult to do, something right to do but something nobody would normally do, and something that others will criticize me for. But in the end I think the voice should not be refused. And so I stopped and stood still, far off to the side of the yurt, near the corner of the altar. I waited, to learn.

Yet still there was silence. Uncle had glanced back down at the book he was teaching, as if to collect his thoughts again. There was a nervous rustle among the boys, and he looked up, and then over at me. His eyes and his voice changed, to something stern, and he said simply, "You may go now, Friday."

He glanced down again at the book, but I could feel his attention on me. I reddened and looked at the floor. I hesitated, for the briefest moment, in defiance and a growing anger. And then out of respect for Uncle I made my way along the altar to the back of the yurt, towards the door.

But then on the floor, in front of me, there was a holy book, the book that Uncle was teaching. Each young monk had a copy, for each one had first been required to write it out in ornate calligraphy, as practice. I stopped short. I could not pass the book, I could not step over it, for in our country of Tibet—and indeed in all the East—our feet are considered very unclean, and we may not step upon or near a sacred thing on the floor. We never wear shoes in the house, and it was considered an act of deep humility to touch or wash another person's feet, as some great saints would do. I could not go on.

I glanced to the side and saw who had put his book there—it was the biggest boy in the class. I knew his name, it was Drom, and there was a bad feeling about him all the time. He looked up with a sneer, and for a moment I stared into his face— the slightly crooked nose, the teeth sharp and mean, like a rat's. I turned and faced Uncle, clutching the churn to my little chest, ready to cry.

His eyes shot up again. "Friday," he said firmly. "Go now. You must go now." My heart was ready to break. Uncle was so good to us. Uncle understood everything, Uncle would not refuse me something only because I was a girl. "I... I..." I stuttered, and closed my eyes hard, and a tear sprang out. I bent my head down to hide it.

And a hand tapped my ankle, and I opened my eyes and looked down. It was Tenzing, leaning behind the big boy, and he silently slid the precious little book out of my path.

I was released, a little bird released. I ran to the door. I whirled around. I felt all the boys' eyes on me, and Uncle's. *I will learn,* I mouthed, silently, and stood up tall and proud in the sunlight at the door. And then I left them.

5.

Showing Adults the Way

The incident with Uncle's tea pushed me over some kind of threshold. I felt an intense yearning to learn what Tenzing and the other boys were learning; even just hearing the bit from Uncle had left me spellbound for days, wondering what kind of idea could protect you, the way a big friend or a sword would protect you, from something very dangerous. But even at that young age I sensed the hopelessness of my quest; even at that age I could feel myself surrounded by the great currents of the mighty river of the-way-things-have-always-been, flowing from centuries before, pushing and pressuring me to grow up as a woman, like Amala and Grandmother Tara, sitting quietly in a darkened yurt, working for a lifetime over a rug or a meal, barred without really noticing it from the door of the world that Tenzing and his friends were already entering. No, I decided, I will not be like that. I will do what girls do not do, whether they want me to or not.

My first step was clear. Tenzing, like all the boys at the nearby monastery, spent the time after our evening meal outside, pacing slowly in a great circle around the family yurts, practicing the books he must commit to memory if he ever hoped to become a Geshe. These books had been written many centuries before in the Mother Tongue, and translated into Tibetan by the first of our country's Lotsawas—the Master Translators. The books were in poetry, to make them easier to memorize, but written in a kind of shorthand or code that your teacher had to explain to you before it could be understood. And so no one else usually paid much attention to the young men as they strolled the monastery grounds, chanting ancient unintelligible wisdom.

But the chants were themselves a thing of great beauty, a different tune for each household of monks, a different melody from each master Teacher. For it was said that there were unseen spirits wandering the world as dusk fell, and that they were sad and tormented, and that—if you sang your book out loudly as you walked—they could hear it and be comforted.

I made my plan as I have always done—a way, in my own mind at least, to trick the world into letting me do something that it didn't normally let people do, but something that would indeed help the world itself if it could be done. I had already decided that the world needed its first Geshe who was a girl. We were after all much different from the boys—I'm not saying necessarily smarter, although that may well be the case—and if boy Geshes can teach and help people with what they've learned, well, then girl Geshes can do the same thing, but with a girl's special touch. And so I knew I had to stake myself out near the stupa.

A stupa, if you do not already know, is a sort of little temple, built almost anywhere—it could be in the middle of a big city, or just by the side of the road somewhere. It's not like people go inside to pray though or anything like that—in fact, you usually can't get inside. The inside is just a little box or something with a very special little object inside it. It might be, oh, say, an old tooth from a very especially kind person who lived long ago, or maybe a little piece of their clothing.

And they just shut it up in there and build the stupa around it—maybe a big onion-shaped dome, or if it was in the countryside just a big pile of stones. Our stupa was like that—it was out back of our family yurt, a huge cairn of rocks that had actually been pulled up when the fields around the house were first cleared. And then Uncle and Father and some of the caravan men had worked hard and built them up into a beautiful peaked shape with a deep niche in the front.

There was a lovely bronze statue of Tara, the Lady of Freedom, sitting upon a flat white stone way in the back; Father had brought it from Nepal. You could stoop in there, and we would often set a few butter lamps on the stone at night. The niche protected them from the wind, and a cheerful light would stream from deep within the stones.

I don't honestly know what the sacred thing sealed inside our stupa was; Uncle said it was something very special he'd brought from the holy land, from India, long ago—but wouldn't say what it was. Not knowing though just made the stupa even more special for Tenzing and me, and we often played near it.

The important thing for me at the moment was that the stupa had been built quite close to the corner of the cattle pen, so you had to go right past it if you wanted to walk around the yurts, or get to the path that led out the back way—the short-cut to the monastery. You see we believe that if you walk around a holy place—whether it be a stupa or your teacher's house—then if you have the right frame of mind and think kind thoughts about people while you go, the blessing of the place will rub off a bit on you, and help you become a better person.

Needless to say, Tenzing—as he chanted the books I was determined to swipe from him—would always be circling around the family yurt and by the stupa. Then he'd go back along the path to our clearing, along the inside of the cattle pen, to Uncle's yurt—because Uncle, for some reason, had insisted on setting his place up right on the edge of the pen. I didn't see how he could sleep with all the noise the animals made, bellowing loudly to each other far into the night, and then again long before daybreak.

Anyway, I'd be able to hear about half of what Tenzing was chanting, and I could repeat it to myself before he doubled back around our yurt for his next round. It wasn't an ideal way to learn, but it was the only way I had. And having a hardship that you know you have to beat sometimes makes you learn a thing better than people who just get it handed to them. So you can say I was lucky.

"Grandmother Tara," I said demurely, setting the first stage of my trap, "will you tell me the story about your name again, about Tara?"

"Of course, child," she replied, and that was already good enough for a few pieces of dried cheese. I sucked on the first and Grandmother was off and running. "You see, if you pray for a long time, and be good for a long time, then you turn into a—well, sort of angel. And then you can go like to three places at once..."

"*Three?*" I said, disbelievingly, to make my little trap more believable.

"Yes, three!" she said. "You could be in the village there, in Kishong; and then be at the monastery, Gempil Ling, too; and still be sitting here in the yurt listening to your grandmother," she concluded, with a knowing nod.

"Why would you want to be in three places at once?" I asked with big round eyes.

"So you could help more people, of course," she replied. "You could be in the village playing with a lonely child, and then over at the monastery on a big occasion like tomorrow evening, helping to light the butter lamps, and still be back here watching the cows for Amala."

I thought for a moment. "But wouldn't that be a little scary? Wouldn't people get upset after a while, and think you were strange?"

"Oh, exactly right," she answered with a nod. "So you go looking like three different people, whatever makes people more comfortable. To the child you make yourself look like another child. To the monks you look like a monk. And maybe here you look like a beautiful grown-up lady."

"And can people learn to do that?" I asked.

"Of course," said Grandmother. "Everyone can learn to do that, and learn to help more and more people, all at the same time. That's what the books are all about; that's why Uncle is teaching people; that's why boys learn to become Geshes. And to remind everybody that sometimes it's more helpful if an Awakened One shows themselves as a girl, well, Tara came into the world—a Buddha who looks like a woman."

"What does your name mean?" I said. "What does Tara mean?"

"It means the Lady of Freedom—the lady who shows people how to be free," she said proudly.

"Who gave you that name?" I persisted.

"Oh," she said, "no one gave it to me. I just decided I liked it and took it when I married your grandfather..." She paused for a moment, sadly.

"I loved the meaning, and I wanted to try to fit into his people, so I took one of their names."

"Then what is your real name?"

"My real name is Tengrar Yowh."
"Does it have a meaning too?"

"In our language, in the Northern Lands, it means Lady of the Sky. In fact, it's the same name as your aunt had, except hers was in the Mother Tongue, and they called her Dakini."

"Dakini…" I said the name, and something struck within my heart. "Dakini. Oh, Grandmother, what was she like? Did you know her?"

"Oh no, child. That was long ago, when your father was still a boy," she said, a little serious.

"That what?" I pried. "Where is she? How come I can't see her?"

"Oh I don't know," replied Grandmother, and I knew it must really be secret, if even Grandmother couldn't find out. "No one really knows, and your Uncle never speaks of it," she said quietly.

I nodded, and saw it was time to get to the stupa. "So if I prayed a lot to Tara, do you think I could learn to be like that—I mean, be in three different places at once, to help people?"

"Of course," said Grandmother Tara, I think happy for my interest in her namesake. "There is even a special prayer, that girls are allowed to learn—it might take you a while, but I think you could even memorize the whole thing. It has 21 different verses, that you sing to her."

"Oh wonderful!" I exclaimed. "Can you teach it to me? And then I could go out maybe in the evenings, to the stupa, and sing it to her there!"

Grandmother paused a bit, I think calculating how long it would take her to get the prayer out of Uncle and learn it herself, and then said brightly, "Of course I can do that. And I'll let Amala and Father know about our little plan, and I'm sure they'll love it. We'll start on the first verse next week, and then do maybe a verse every few weeks, if that's not too much. Can you manage that, little girl?" she beamed.

I beamed back and stood up on the bed and hugged her around the neck. Then one last thing occurred to me. "What's the big occasion at the monastery tomorrow, Grandmother?"

"It's the enthronement of the new abbot, or actually the old abbot, but anyway it's quite a sight. And your father is planning a big bonfire afterwards, to celebrate," she said, gazing at me with her little-girl eyes. "And yes, of course, you and I will go together."

I squealed with delight, more over the fact that I had been able to coax this particularly stubborn adult into my trap so successfully. It was just like leading one of the friendlier cows out to the pasture on a rope.

That evening I went to tidy up Tara's altar, at the stupa. She looked at me a little sternly, but I think she approved. Tenzing strolled by, just starting to sing the first line of his first book:

Those who listen, seeking peace...

I did listen, and right there I began. In time, Grandmother Tara was able to teach me the whole song to Tara, the 21 verses. But by the time I was ten years old, Tenzing—and I—had finished memorizing the three most important books of the Geshe course: over a thousand verses. And no one but my own heart ever heard me sing them.

6.

The Lady of the Throne

Grandmother Tara and I approached the main temple of the monastery of Gempil Ling. If you have never been to such a temple on a great feast day, it's a little hard to know what it feels like. Every single monk from our monastery—and everyone from the whole countryside around—was there, dressed in his finest golden robes; they overflowed out the great lacquered doorways onto the porch and steps, sitting on the ground on cushions, in rows facing each other. On a day like this everyone was allowed to wear the tall pointed hat of a Geshe, and these waved in a great sea as the monks chanted prayers of good tidings in unison, swaying in union to the beat of the great drums. The walls of every building around, and the ground itself, shook with their rhythm.

Villagers jammed the aisles up the steps and into the temple, where they filed quietly along the great stone walls, behind the singing monks, to the altars, to make a prayer and offer a lamp. Somewhere in there, crushed among the junior monks, would be Tenzing and his classmates; even Uncle had been coaxed out of his yurt for the occasion, and would be sitting up near the front, with the senior Geshes.

We stepped towards the threshold of the temple. The chant was reaching a great crescendo, with hundreds of voices straining for the highest notes. A great warm wind full of the warmth of human bodies, and the fragrance of incense, and the smell of the butter burning in thousands of tiny lamps, struck my face. A line of about ten high Lamas, in special hats and elaborate robes, was making its way in a solemn procession straight up the middle of the sea of sound and humanity. I stood balanced on the threshold of the massive temple doors. Grandmother stepped ahead, holding my hand. But I couldn't move.

She was on the throne. I could see her over the line of golden hats, and she was golden too, but more golden, because she was golden light itself. She looked up then, and her eyes met mine. They were strange eyes, full of love, but power too.

I broke away from Grandmother. She called but I could not have heard. I ran straight for the

Lady on the throne. Straight down the center of all the monks. I had to reach her. I had to touch her. Past the flowing silks of the high Lamas. Over the delicate symbols of goodness painted on the floor before the altar. Up the hard-packed clay steps to the throne, and then reaching for her, hands outstretched, arms and heart thrown up to her, trying to get up the wooden steps of the throne itself.

She gazed down at me, and I saw her then clearly, and she smiled to say that all was well, and that the time would come—and then there were strong hands grasping me under the arms, hoisting me back to the floor at the side of the throne.

"Whoa there, little girl!" said a big monk with a great smiling face. "That seat's already taken today, unless you happen to be the new abbot of Gempil Ling!"

I looked up at him in excitement and pointed to the Lady already there on the throne, but she was gone. I frowned in confusion and clutched the happy monk's huge warm hand.

"What's all this about, Geshe Lothar?" I heard a cheerful voice behind me, over the din. I turned and saw that the procession of Lamas had reached the altar, and the throne. The monk in front was a short, rounded, jolly man with a big grin and slightly crossed eyes, warmth pouring out of him.

"I don't know, Precious One," replied the monk who had caught me. "But it looks like you might have some competition for your new job," he smiled. Then the Precious One took my other little hand in his, and bent down close to my face with a quizzical look. He pinched me happily on the cheek, and said "Hi there," and straightened back up.

"There's no way you're going to get her safely out of this crush right now," he said, looking back over the mass of chanting monks and crowds of villagers. "I suggest you just sit her down and keep her with you through to the end of the ceremony—whoever lost her has surely seen her by now, and will show up to fetch her afterwards." And then I noticed that nearly every face below was turned up towards us, necks craning, trying to see what was going on and why a little girl was up disrupting the installment of the next Abbot of Gempil Ling.

The Precious One, the Abbot, turned and ascended the steps to the throne. To each side of this central throne, where the Lady had been sitting, were several other thrones—lower—for former abbots of the monastery and visiting dignitaries. The Lama up on the throne to the right stood out from the others, a little like a boy version of Grandmother, with a high aristocratic neck and an aura of authority. He turned his eyes down at me coldly, with a look of disapproval, and despite myself I shivered a bit. But then the happy monk, Geshe Lothar, had already pulled me down next to him into a row of kindly-looking older monks— right up on the platform before the altars, which consisted of great stone slabs that stretched across the whole front of the temple.

"What's wrong, little one?" he whispered loudly with a smile, leaning his head over near mine in the noise. I looked up at him.

"That other Lama, on the other throne. He looks so mean!" I whispered back.

Geshe Lothar looked across and then back to me. "Oh him," he said slowly. "That's the Founding Father himself! The one who started this whole monastery, many years ago; the first of our abbots, and still mostly the real boss around here, no matter who they call the Abbot. And he's not really mean," said Geshe Lothar, and paused, "just tough. You have to be tough, to start a new place like this, in a country where there's never really been a lot of monasteries before now."

"Oh," I said. And then I caught the eye of the Abbot, the monk they called Precious One. His throne, which in our temples is really just a fancy cushion up on a very high narrow platform, had a funny little table next to it, with skinny little legs almost as tall as a man. And there was a monk with a great brass pitcher reaching up as high as he could, pouring fresh Tibetan tea into a delicate white Chinese porcelain cup on the table. The Precious One winked at me, and pointed to the tea, and then to me as if to say, "You're going to get some too!"

"But *he* looks like a really nice man," I said to Geshe Lothar, pointing with my head to the Abbot.

"Oh, the Precious One... he is, he really is. Got to have a strong heart and a great sense of humor to be Abbot of this place, or any other big monastery. You see, monks are very stubborn people—you have to be stubborn to stay a monk— and to run a big group of them you have to be a wise and patient man. Now the Precious One, Geshe Donyo, he's just that. And humble and funny on top of it, so everybody likes him. That's why the monks have chosen him to be abbot for another six years, and that's what we're all celebrating today."

He stopped and gave me a long look in the eyes. "Would you like to be an Abbot, little one?" he laughed.

"Oh, yes," I said. "All the fancy robes he gets to wear, and everybody has to listen to him, and he gets his tea first before anyone else." I pointed out to the crowd, where novices bearing even larger pitchers of tea were working through the rows of monks. Each monk pulled a small wooden bowl out from under his robes, to receive a portion, and held it steaming in his palms, on his lap.

"Ah that," laughed Geshe Lothar. "Now think about it a bit more carefully before you say that," he laughed again. "That pile of special robes on top of the Abbot is really hot and uncomfortable, especially up near the roof like that. Can't you see him sweating?" he giggled. I looked up, and saw it was so, and giggled back.

"And as far as telling everyone what to do— that's his job, and that's what he does, but nobody listens any more than they absolutely have to. It's a very hard position to be in," he said, with a knowing nod.

"And as for the tea," he whispered finally, for the temple had suddenly quieted down to a nearly complete silence. "They give him that fancy little cup, but it doesn't hold much more tea than a thimble would. And he does get served first, but then he has to wait for the very last baby little monk out there somewhere at the bottom of the front steps to get his share, before he can start the grace over the tea. And by that time the Abbot's tea is ice cold and hardly fit to drink. I bet he'd rather have that baby monk's big hot bowlful any day." Geshe Lothar grinned, and leaned back up with a serious official look, as someone next to him pushed a bowl of tea into his own hands. After a while the Precious One started up a grace, and everyone chanted along, and offered the first sip to the Awakened Ones.

Then there was a long meal, with young monks running up and down the aisles and serving everybody ceremonial rice with raisins and little brown roots, like truffles, that tasted like nuts. This they carried in huge wicker baskets, and ladled out into the same wooden bowls. Then everyone, including all the villagers, got a huge round piece of sweetened flatbread, baked in the monastery kitchen that morning on huge skillets made of massive sheets of slate from the ridge of stone near our home. Then finally everyone was given a special treat—a cup of tea with milk and a generous dollop of precious sugar in it.

As people enjoyed their food, the Chanting Master—a big fat monk with a deep loud booming voice that matched his tummy—got up and stood quite close to us. He unrolled a long scroll and bellowed out some long proclamation about the new abbot and other monastery officers—I don't remember exactly how it went, because I was getting very tired from all the excitement, the heat in the temple, and the goodies that Geshe Lothar kept pressing on me, like some big jolly version of Amala.

And then at the end each of the monks tossed the last few pieces of his flatbread out on the floor in front of him, and tucked his bowl back under his robes. A final wave of novices rushed in and trotted up and down the rows, dropping a small hand-broom made of reeds in front of every third or fourth monk. With these the monks reached out and swept the pieces of bread towards the back of the temple, where again novices appeared with huge baskets. All the bits of bread were piled into these—some were taken out to the surrounding fields and emptied, as a gift to all the little creatures and spirits who shared our land with us. Other baskets were carried up to the roof of the temple, and set out for the great ravens and falcons that we saw as protectors of our monastery and village. They would be waiting, circling in a huge spiral flock that towered hundreds of feet into the sky of deepest blue, tinged crimson now with the setting of the sun.

Finally the Precious One cleared his throat and announced the final chant of the day, the opening pages of the first of the Five Great Books of the Geshe course. I turned towards Geshe Lothar and whispered loudly, *"Those who listen, seeking peace."* His jaw dropped in amazement; I didn't bother to tell him that all I knew was the first half of the first line, or that I had only just learned it the night before.

And then as the chanting started up once more, the Abbot came back down the steps of his throne, and led the procession of high Lamas again—this time up past the thrones to the altar itself, with its huge statues of holy beings and wonderful teachers of centuries gone by. When they passed us, Geshe Lothar stood and lifted me up by my hand again, and we fell into line right behind the Abbot and the Founding Father. Suddenly it dawned on me that this big happy monk was himself one of the highest of the Lamas of Gempil Ling.

We stepped up to each of the beautiful statues, in the bright golden light of the butter lamps, and stopped to offer each peaceful figure a white ceremonial scarf called a *kata*. These can be over ten feet long and are a universal symbol of welcome and friendship throughout our land; as we stepped down to the floor of the temple, villagers pushed forth, thrusting huge piles of the soft white silk into the arms of the new Abbot. He paused before each joyful smile and, according to tradition, returned each scarf to the person who had offered it, hanging it around their bowed neck and touching their heads in his warm palms as a blessing.

It was a custom for the high Lamas to leave the temple down the very last aisle, off to the side, through the rows of very beginning monks. I walked in sort of a full and happy daze behind Geshe Lothar, holding his hand. It happened when we were almost to the doors of the temple.

As we passed some of the young monks I saw a flash out of the corner of my eye, and then I fell on something. My hand slipped out of Geshe Lothar's, and I scraped my knee badly on the floor. I cried out and Geshe Lothar spun around to pick me up. One of the small hand-brooms was lying on the floor under me. He picked this up in his other hand and straightened up slowly, sternly, staring at a little huddle of three novices in the row nearby.

I looked up and followed his eye and saw the three—the one in the middle, I suddenly realized, was my brother's classmate: the big one, Drom. He had a defiant smile plastered across his face, and his eyes rose and challenged Geshe Lothar's. The big happy monk suddenly looked different, strong and righteous, but then he just paused, and looked up the line of Lamas and attendants—they had all paused, and were looking back at us. The Founding Father stared for a moment, and Geshe Lothar's eyes dropped to the floor.

The Precious One bent his neck and looked out almost through his eyebrows, in a way he had, with his crossed eyes and like a true Abbot, he grasped the entire incident in a single glance. Then he reached out to the Founding Father and took him by the arm and pulled him along, with a big funny smile and a "Wonderful ceremony, was it not?"

7.

Fire and Alarm

Grandmother Tara was waiting by the threshold of the temple with a look of sheer anger in her eyes. As Geshe Lothar and I stepped on to the porch she grasped me by the arm and pulled me to her side. Geshe Lothar glanced at her face only an instant, and knew exactly what to say.

"Oh, so you must be the proud mother of this amazing little girl!" he boomed at Grandmother.

"Well, actually, her grandmother," she tittered, with a growing smile. "And you are...?"

"Geshe Lothar, Giku of Gempil Ling: Vice-Abbot and Debate Master, at your service!" he answered, as masses of monks and villagers began to stream past us, out the doorways, into the courtyard. "And I can tell you that this little girl is smart as a whip, and had us all quite amazed, and will grow up into someone quite special if she gets a chance!" he gushed.

Grandmother opened her mouth to begin telling Geshe Lothar about how it was all in the family blood, but he seemed to see it coming, and blurted out, "Well, good to see her back safe with you! Got to run now; you know, first official meeting of the new monastery officers and the Council of Elders starts right away, upstairs!" He pointed his arm up a flight of stairs at the end of the porch, and bent down to squeeze my hand with a big smile, and flew off in a flutter of ceremonial robes.

"See you again soon!" he yelled over his shoulder, giving me a quick wink.

"A true gentleman!" exclaimed Grandmother, cooled down considerably. Then she turned to the front steps of the temple porch and led me through the milling crowd of monks and villagers to the trunk of a tree near the low wall around the temple.

"I told Tenzing to meet us here," said Grandmother firmly. "I knew it would be almost dark by the time we got out of there, and we'd never find him otherwise in this crowd. Then we'll be off to the bonfire. Your uncle is going to be stuck in that same meeting for a while, and said he'd meet up with us later."

We stood and waited, and people filed out the little gate next to us. Several matrons from the village nodded at Grandmother, eyes running up and down her fine holiday outfit. One large lady that I recognized as the keeper of a small tea shop on the horse road not far from our place stopped and gave me a long surprised look, and said to Grandmother, "Why, she got to be right up there in front with the high Lamas, the whole time!" And Grandmother nodded proudly and began to trace our family line back again and my brother Tenzing rushed up in his handsome dress robes and grasped me by the arms.

"Friday! I can't believe you did that!" he hissed, in a voice of awe mixed with embarrassment. "Whatever came over you? What was the Vice-Abbot saying to you all that time? And..." he lowered his voice "... how mad is Grandmother Tara?"

I glanced over at the two spinsters, now chattering away with ooh's and ah's, and gazed up at the official suites in the highest floors of the temple, thanking Geshe Lothar. Then I turned my face up to Tenzing's and announced, "Grandmother is very pleased. Geshe Lothar is a true gentleman. And I had a reason to be up in front, and it's none of your business." I giggled and kicked him in the shin, and he looked down at my bloodied knee. His face tensed darkly.

"I saw who did that..." he began, but then Grandmother was pulling us along with one arm while she waved the other for emphasis to a growing crowd of older ladies who were headed our way, and anxious to hear my story. I had become a minor celebrity by the time we got out of the monastery walls and onto the horse road.

"You know," Grandmother was saying, "her uncle is an old friend of the Abbot, and practically his right-hand man." Tenzing turned his face to me as we walked, and rolled his eyes. "And our family is particularly close to Geshe Lothar, who—as you probably know—is the Vice-Abbot and Debate Master." This time it was my turn to roll my eyes. Then as everyone settled into walking and talking we got free of Grandmother and dropped back a ways. The ceremony had been scheduled for the full moon, and it was rising over the mountains to the east, flooding the road in a soft light.

"It was Drom," said Tenzing grimly. "As you and the Lamas started down the aisle, I saw him and his two buddies cooking up some plan, but I didn't realize what it was—and I was stuck two rows back on the other side and couldn't have gotten out anyway. Then just as you walked by he slid the broom out under your feet."

"But why?" I asked.

"Oh, he's just mean," said Tenzing, with a scowl, "and he doesn't like it when other people get attention. He's always acting up in class, and him and Stick and Hammer are always giving me a hard time, because they think I'm the teacher's pet."

"Who's Stick and Hammer?" I asked.

"Oh, the two boys that hang out with him— the two you saw with him today. I guess there was a mean king back in India in the old days, and he squeezed his subjects to give him everything they had, and whenever they didn't give enough he'd send his two evil ministers to punish them, and after a while the people named them Stick and Hammer, because that's what they'd use to hit people when they didn't give enough. And so Drom uses those names for the other two guys in his gang, because he likes to think of himself like a big King who can use his Stick and Hammer to hurt us other boys. Stick is the tall thin one that never smiles—Hammer is the chubby one with the mean laugh.

"And you really have to keep out of their way, Friday," he concluded seriously, stopping in the road and taking my hands.

I looked up with my stubborn look and said, "I don't have to keep out of anybody's way, Tenzing."

"But they might start picking on you if you don't," he said with concern.

"Doesn't matter to me!" I raised my voice.

"They can do really bad stuff," he warned.

"I don't care, I'm not afraid to tell if they do something!" I shot back.

"Um… it's kind of hard to tell on them," replied Tenzing. "Everyone's afraid of Drom's uncle, and he gets away with almost anything."

"Doesn't matter to me!" I repeated. "I'd tell Uncle Jampa!" And then I got an idea and said, "I could even tell the Abbot, and get him in a lot of trouble!" Then I got really inspired. "I'd even tell on Drom to the Founding Father himself, if I had to!" I squawked.

"I don't think so," said Tenzing glumly, and started walking down the road again.

"And why not?" I yelled ahead at him, stamping my foot.

Tenzing turned back. "Because the Founding Father," he said quietly, "is who Drom's uncle is."

I looked down at the ground in frustration and suddenly understood why Geshe Lothar and everyone else had acted so strangely after I fell. I couldn't believe it.

But there was nothing to do about it tonight, and just then I caught sight of the bonfire, still a good half hour's walk away, and ran to catch up with Tenzing.

Father had purchased a good-sized field on the side of the horse road quite a distance from home. The crops had been taken in a few weeks before, and the caravan men—who were just back from a long trip to Nepal—had gathered all the dried stubble together and thrown on some huge logs for a wonderful fire. Father had ordered huge kettles of tea and a Mongolian-style stew called *lauvsha* that he knew Grandmother especially would enjoy, and was treating everyone on the holiday. All the caravan men's families were there too—the women had brought big bowl-shaped metal skillets with long handles on each side,

71

together with sacks of ground barley. They always took advantage of a bonfire to stand and roast the barley flour into *sampa*, a favorite staple in our country. People would throw a few spoonfuls into a bowl and pour in some buttered Tibetan tea and mix it up into a delicious pasty stuff. It was especially popular with the monks who went for months or years to a cave, to pray and meditate.

At the fire, a person would stand on each side and grab a handle. Then they'd sweep the skillet over the flames, swinging the barley up into the air on each pass so it wouldn't burn, and catching it again in the skillet as it flew down, for the next pass over the fire. They'd sing beautiful old barley songs from long ago, and everyone around the fire would sit and listen, and sing along if they knew the tune. It was a way that we had, to make work into a really fun time. Later on people would even start to dance by the fire, and Grandmother would always get up at least once and do a Northern dance that began with her arms flung out straight to the sides and a slow stamp with her feet, and then (depending on how inspired she felt) would find her spinning furiously with her head thrown back and laughing.

Tenzing and I employed our usual trick to get away from the adults. We ran breathlessly up to Grandmother, who was still haranguing a few tired listeners about our family history. We told her we'd be with Father and Amala, and she waved goodbye distractedly. Then we ran around to the other side of the fire and found Father and Amala. Father was busy as usual, directing the feeding of all the people like a great military campaign, and Amala was at his side, quiet but looking happy for once, and it was really good to see. She rubbed Tenzing's head affectionately and we blurted out that we'd be with Grandmother; and she just smiled and nodded and looked back to the arrangements.

Tenzing and I knew right where to go. Off to the side away from the road there'd be a little cluster of the old-timers, caravan hands who had ridden with Grandfather himself. They'd have a little fire going and be passing around a jug of *chang*. This was some kind of mild brew of alcohol—I tasted it once, it was a little like pear juice but had a bitter taste mixed in with it. Father was a sincere Buddhist and disapproved of drinking, but left the old-timers to their ways if they kept it to themselves. Anyway Tenzing and I really liked to hang out with them, because they told the best stories.

One of them, a real original with hollowed cheeks and only a few teeth left in his mouth, was already going strong on our favorite subject, the *Dremo:* the one you call the Yeti, or the Abominable Snowman. He was getting to the good part, with a wicked gleam in his eye, glinting red from the flames of the larger bonfire.

"And so there we was, standing knee-deep in the snow at the pass, and this big feller—must'a been fifteen foot at least—starts running down this hill at us, all huge and white and fur and fangs." He caught sight of Tenzing and me, and opened his mouth wide to stick out a lonely front tooth for emphasis.

We gasped and pulled up closer and exclaimed, "What did you do then?"

"Well of course we grabs the paddles out of our packs and starts slapping out the *zadak*," he replied, taking a swig from a nearby jug.

"What's a *zadak*?" we cried back in unison.

"Oh! *Zadak*!" he belched, but we didn't move back much because we really wanted to know.

"Sort of like, an alarm, you see," he said, squinting as though he was having a little trouble seeing us. "You takes two big flat sticks and you slaps 'em together a special way and holler like crazy, and even if people can't hear you yellin' they hear the slappin' 'cause that sound carries nearly a mile up high, like we is here," he explained, and then lost the thread of his story while he gazed around for the jug, which had travelled on.

"Well what does the *zadak* sound like?" we insisted.

"Why, it's always the same," he replied, turning back to us with a distracted look, and he raised his hands and made a soft clap. "One beat," he said, "and then a pause. Then two beats," he clapped twice again, "and another pause, while you yells *Zadak! Danger!* at the top of your lungs. Then just start over and keep goin' for dear life, until somebody shows up to help, or the critter eats ya alive, whichever comes first!" he wheezed.

"Did he eat you?" we chorused.

"Well, no," replied the old-timer, looking a little abashed. "Can't say as he did. He just up and runs straight on through the caravan line, chasing after a *cheebee,* and we never laid eyes on him again."

"What's a *chee—bee*?" we chorused again.

"*Cheebee*?" he said dumbly, gazing around for the little jug again. "*Cheebee*? Oh, that'd be a little groundhog, lives up near the top of the mountains."

"Did he eat the *cheebee*?" another chorus.

The old-timer tried to lay his eyes back on us. "Well no," he muttered. "They rarely eats them, after all."

"Why not?"

"Well 'cause you see them snow monsters, they only likes to eat in the evening. And the *cheebees,* well, they only comes out in the middle of the day. So when a snow monster sees a *cheebee* he just grabs hold o' them and sits right down on top o' him and waits till evening comes, so's he can have him all fresh and warm like, ya see."

"And then do they eat them?" final chorus.

"Well no," he said, with a sly smile. "That's the whole point, don't ya see, why he ran right past us without so much as a blink. 'Cause every time a snow monster is sittin' on one *cheebee* he goes and sees another one runnin' around and so he jumps up to get that one and the first one gets away and pretty soon those little guys got that big monster runnin' every which way, and nobody gets eated at all!"

"Yay!" we cried happily, and the old-timer cackled with pleasure. Then Tenzing and I jumped up and ran right into the dark, away from the fires, down the road—to practice making the *zadak* ourselves.

Tenzing found a couple of big sticks and pounded out the beats while I did the yelling, but I was careful to face away from the bonfire. They were all singing loud anyway and we figured no one would hear us. It was the most fun, and we were jabbering on at each other about how we'd probably get a snow monster to show up, when we heard the strangest noise.

"Stop it Friday! Stop!" cried Tenzing. "Listen to that!" I stopped yelling and listened. I don't know if you've ever heard a sound like that, like you're sitting quietly on a really still day, in a place out in the middle of nowhere that has some trees around, and suddenly—very far away—you hear a sort of a low roar, and then it gets louder and louder, and then a really strong gust of wind rips across you—the wind racing towards you through the trees. And that was the sound, and we waited scared for a few moments, to see what would hit us.

And then there in the moonlight it was just Uncle; we knew and loved him well and could tell his silhouette anywhere—and he stepped forward upon us urgently.

"Tenzing! Friday! What are you doing? Why are you making the *zadak*? What's happened?"

Tenzing froze with the two sticks in his hand, and I stared down at the ground. Uncle knew then it was a false alarm; he stooped and grabbed us each by an arm. "Listen, you two. There's a rule about the *zadak*. People only make it when there's a real emergency, like someone has seen a snow leopard prowling near the houses, or maybe even some bandits on horseback headed for the village. But children," he squeezed our arms for emphasis, "are never allowed to make the *zadak*. You were lucky it was me coming up the road from the monastery, and not someone else—or you'd really be in big trouble by now. Do you understand?" he finished forcefully.

Tenzing nodded quietly but suddenly the whole long day was just too much for me, and I started bawling. Uncle sat still for a minute to let the scolding sink in and then stood up, and smiled. He took each of us by the hand, and I wondered as always at how hot his hand seemed, even outside in the cold. And then soon we were sitting by the big fire again, one on each side of Uncle, and he had an arm around each of us, in a big hug. He watch my last few tears roll down, and then reached into his shoulderbag and fished out something wrapped in a cloth.

"This might fix you two up," he grinned, and unfolded the cloth, to reveal—bugs.

"*Boolook*!" cried Tenzing and I, together.

"That's right," said Uncle. "There was a big pile of them put out on the altar, and when the Temple Keeper and his crew cleaned up, they brought some up to our meeting to pass around. Sort of a reward for not falling asleep while people take hours to make a few simple decisions," he sighed. Then he held up a big piece, and broke it in two, and gave us each half to chew on.

But I mean, if you don't know, they're not really bugs. That's just what we call them: *boolook*, or deep-fried bugs. Really you just get a big pot of butter boiling a bit, and then you take like a sock (but one that you've just washed, you know) and poke a little hole in the toe (if there's not one there already). Then you pour a few cups of sweet flour batter into the sock, and hold it over the pot of butter while you squeeze it (just a touch) and then the batter comes out in a little stream and you wave the sock around and little squiggles form all over each other on the top of the butter. They look like little bugs all stuck together, and then when it gets nice and brown you take it out with a big spatula and lay it on a dish and maybe sprinkle a little honey or even sugar on it and then when it cools down enough (or even a little before that) you can eat it—you just break little bugs off—it's the best.

Now Tenzing and I had a rule, I don't remember how it started, but whenever we ate our meals we would always share half of every piece of whatever it was on each of our plates, even though it was exactly the same thing. We just liked sharing everything. It was like we were really just one big person with a single stomach and two mouths. So I broke my bugs in two very solemnly and handed him over half, and he did the same for me. Then we settled down to chewing and watching the fire and listening to the happy songs. I was nearly asleep in the warmth of the fire and Uncle's arm, when he leaned over and whispered to me, "Friday, little Friday."

"Yes Uncle Jampa?" I answered, sleepily.

"Tell me," he said quietly, "tell me... who was it you saw on the throne today, when you ran past all the Lamas, up to the front of the temple?"

Suddenly I felt very happy, because I knew Uncle knew I had seen someone, and I had been afraid to tell anyone so far.

"It was a Lady," I murmured, snuggling into the soft cloth of his monk's shawl. "A golden Lady, all made of light."

Uncle nodded seriously, and stared ahead into the fire for a pretty long time.

And then he said quietly to me, "Friday, little one… her face—did you see her face?"

"Oh yes Uncle," I answered dreamily, just before I fell asleep. "I did, I saw her face. And she had the most special eyes… " I looked up at Uncle and for a moment his eyes looked almost the same. "Like yours," I whispered last—and then I fell into the most beautiful dream, and he picked me up, and carried me all the way home.

8.

The Warriors of Wisdom

It was the following spring I think that Grandmother Tara first took me to see the wisdom warriors. They fought at night, and the old people from all around enjoyed the walk together down the horse road as evening fell, to get out and about, and have a good time together while doing something meaningful at the monastery.

I will never forget that first time. We were still a good quarter mile from the main gates of the monastery; Grandmother was gossiping happily with a few kindly, gray-haired friends. And then I heard the sound, like thunder way off in the distance. As we got closer it grew louder and louder, until by the time we had come to the main gates of the monastery it was difficult for the elders to talk to one another without yelling. We turned downhill just outside the gates and skirted the great wall that circled the monastery. In a few minutes we came to a lower wall, about waist high, set around a huge courtyard. I stopped in my tracks, dumbfounded by the roar, and drank in one of the most astounding sights of my entire life.

There were torches stuck at intervals into the top of the wall, and in their red flickering light I could see over a hundred of the student monks leaping and dancing and twirling in some huge wild rhythm. They flew into the air shouting with glee and then came down on one foot, stamping the ground with the other, like a great bull smashing at the earth with his hoof. Their arms shot up over their heads, swinging a long string of beads, and then one hand came down hard on the other, both thrust out before them, in a thunderous clap. Then they whirled around and ran back a few yards, turned, and launched their bodies forward again, in another leap and shouts of exultation, smashing their hands together with such force that the skin between the fingers split open, little droplets of blood spraying the air in front of them.

And only then I noticed that before each swirling monk there was another monk, just sitting quietly on a thin piece of rug thrown down over the gray flagstones. The sitting monk sat perfectly still, like the Buddha that you see in pictures, sitting below the big tree: rock-solid, unmoving, like a wall that the dancing monk would throw his body into, to see if it would move. And it did not.

I was captivated; the very ground beneath us, and my whole being, sang with the roar of the warriors.

I tugged at Grandmother's silken sleeves excitedly and lifted my face up to hers and cried, "What are they doing, Grandmother! It's so... it's so wonderful!"

Grandmother Tara just stood tall and straight and gazed over the wall impassively, the torchlight catching her regal features. And then she held me close in front of her, so we could both watch, while she yelled near my ear, to be heard.

"They are warriors!" she cried exultantly, and I felt her Northern blood stirring through the strong fingers on my shoulders. "Warriors of wisdom! And this is how they learn their wisdom, in the heat of the battle of the minds!"

I could only nod and stare, in awe. They never stopped, never paused, the whole courtyard flashing in flying red robes, lips gasping for breath, faces on fire with delight and the quest for understanding, sweat pouring down the cheeks and chests and slender rippling arms. I strained to hear the words.

"But what are they saying?" I screamed in excitement, pulling Grandmother right up to the side of the wall.

She threw her head back like a Mongol fighting man and gave a wild laugh that flew into the roar around us as if it were going home. "You and I will never know, little Friday!" she shouted over the noise. And then she leaned over me and said, "Because girls don't do that, you know," and she pointed to the war before us.

I turned back on her violently with my mouth wide open, and the voice came into my head again, and it was louder than a hundred monks, louder even than if they had been dragons; and it covered the courtyard and the monastery and proclaimed, "Girls do do that!" But to Grandmother I just threw a look of fury and determination so loud that her face broke into a great beam and she had to cry out, "Good for you, girl!" Then she reached down and grabbed my hand and fairly skipped away along the wall towards the back of the courtyard. We passed several knots of villagers, leaning over the wall, just staring, and fingering simple prayers on the beads that almost every Tibetan person carries with them all the time. Quite near the back corner, where the monastery fields stretched away from the wall in the dark, we came on a place where the plows had turned a pile of fresh earth up against the stones. We stood there and leaned over the top of the wall.

"Wait," said Grandmother to me firmly. "Watch."

The melee looked different from this end — towards the far wall now I could see a great pavilion, open on four sides, with towering pillars and a Chinese-style pagoda roof. Against the back wall there was a high throne of wood, with steps leading up to it at the side. There in the very center of the pavilion was sort of a high, wide bench. I began to notice that the monks leaping to and fro under and around the pavilion were older, and their movements more practiced and fluid. Here on the side near the fields the monks were younger, about Tenzing's age; they made more noise I think but even I could tell they were just learning the elaborate flying steps and handclaps.

Then off in the light near the pavilion I saw a strong, taller figure emerge from a gateway. He raised one arm under his monk's shawl and waved it back and forth as he stepped forward, shooing the young monks ahead of him, as though he were a mother hen.

"The Debate Master," said Grandmother. "That is, your friend — Geshe Lothar." She spoke in hushed tones, for suddenly the furious battle had subsided to a quiet rustle as the young monks, panting for breath, stopped and walked in small clusters to specific spots around the courtyard.

"That was just the warm-up," said Grandmother, turning her face towards mine. She had a look of excitement, like a little girl, and I suddenly realized why she went out on walks to the monastery so often in the evenings.

"The warriors will sit now with their own classmates, in a group, and then the fun will start again. The older monks get to sit closer to the bright lights and the pavilion—the baby monks get stuck back here," and she nodded with her head to the nearby corner. "We'll be able to see everything," she followed my glance as it darted back to her, "and hear pretty well too," she smiled.

Even as we watched, a group of about fifteen young monks quietly coalesced where Grandmother had pointed. Suddenly I spotted Tenzing, and jabbed Grandmother with an elbow. She gazed towards him steadily, with a look of pride.

The monks squatted in a huddle for a moment. Each unwrapped a special string of beads from his left wrist and threw it into a pile in the middle of the huddle. Then a pleasant-looking but serious young monk grabbed all the beads up in his two palms and threw them high into the air. He closed his eyes and reached up and grabbed one string of beads out of the tangled mass as it fell back to the earth.

This he handed solemnly to its owner—a thin, short novice with big eyes and buck teeth and sort of a frightened look about him.

"What are they doing?" I hissed. I had to know everything.

"The class leader," whispered Grandmother, "has just chosen the defender. And now he repeats the process to select the attacker."

The mass of beads went up again, and this time a tall, powerful form stepped forward to claim his string. With a twinge I saw it was Drom, the trouble-maker.

The little monk stood still for a moment, sizing up his opponent nervously. Then he turned quietly, stepped to the wall of the courtyard, and sat down with his back against it. The big boy, Drom, walked back away from the wall about twenty feet, already staring down at the smaller boy and twisting his beads in his strong hands, as if he were getting ready for a fight.

The class leader sat down in front of the monk at the wall, off to the side a bit. I saw Tenzing step forward resolutely and sit across from him. Then the other boys filled in, two rows deep on either side, facing each other and forming an empty aisle between Drom and the smaller boy. It got very silent and you could feel the tension mounting.

"The attacker prepares," whispered Grandmother with a wicked smile, "in his mind. The defender quiets his heart, and prays to his Teacher for strength."

Then the big boy walked slowly down the aisle between the rows of monks and stopped with his feet only about an inch from the smaller boy's crossed legs. He looked like a bear towering over a mouse, considering whether it was even worth the trouble to eat.

Then the big one—Drom—reached up and removed the corner of his monk's shawl from his shoulder, in an ancient gesture of respect. The small boy on the ground bowed his head.

"The opponents salute each other, and no matter what their feelings may be otherwise, they sincerely pray for each other to succeed in the battle: they pray that both they themselves, and all who listen and watch, may leave at the end of the war with more understanding than they had before."

I looked up at Grandmother with a new respect. She understood and laughed and said, "Oh, I'm not so smart. But I must say this stuff intrigues me. Every once in a while an older monk comes out one of the back gates in the monastery wall," she waved with her head up past the front of the courtyard, to the big wall. "They shut all the gates pretty early, but they built the courtyard of the wisdom warriors outside the main wall, so village people could come and watch, even at night. They say even just hearing a little of what is spoken here puts a good seed in your mind for the future, even for after you die.

"I don't know about all that," Grandmother mused then, "but as you know I am fairly curious," she laughed. "So anyway when an older monk needs to pee-pee at night you see they come out the gate and walk past here out to the fields somewhere, and on the way back we stop them and ask them to explain to us a little about what's going on, and that's how I learned." Then she raised her head back to Tenzing's class.

The big boy straightened and replaced his shawl, then leaned over and cried out "Di!" in a high-pitched voice.

"What's that?" I whispered urgently, my heart stopping.

"It is a word from the Mother Tongue, from Sanskrit," explained Grandmother, looking at the boys intently. "It is part of an ancient prayer that people use to ask the Awakened One for understanding—and it means 'wisdom.' It is also," she stared in obvious anticipation, "the call to battle."

Suddenly the big boy leaped up into the air, and screamed at the top of his lungs a string of words, fast, like arrows from a dozen bows at once. I caught only one phrase—it was *ten ching drelwar jungwa na*. My breath caught in my throat, my heart leaped over the wall into the air between the two warriors. I knew those words. It was part of what Tenzing sang every night as he passed me at the altar of the little stupa shrine. It was part of what I had learned to sing after him, in silence. But I had no idea what it meant.

I strained to hear. The words flying from the big boy's mouth whipped past my ears and out into the dark night behind us, a confusion of birds fluttering in a flock when someone has thrown a stone at them.

"What is he saying?" I cried again at Grandmother.

She looked down at me in obvious sympathy, and then back at the leaping monk. She squinted her eyes for a moment in concentration and then turned back to face me, slowly. "Oh little Friday," she said, louder now, as battles began to break out in each one of the groups scattered about the courtyard. "I don't really know. You see it is all very old words, from very old books—close even to the Mother Tongue itself. And then in the middle they throw in some regular talk, like 'What's that mean?' or 'Do you really think that?'

"All I know for sure is what they told me—that the attacker pulls out say one important sentence from the old book they're working on, and first he sees if the defender can even remember where it's from. They can't bring any books along with them, you see—it all has to be in their mind. And that's why," she said, with a bit of condescension that rattled me, "your brother Tenzing walks around singing those books over and over again every evening, to get them into his mind, firmly." I opened my mouth, but then just closed it. Even at that age I knew when not to know.

"Then the attacker, he says something about that little sentence, that one little idea. But he purposely says something that's just a tiny bit wrong. And then the defender has to try to figure out what the attacker said that was a little bit wrong, and prove it was wrong, in front of everybody. Here comes the wrong idea right now!" she cried. The big boy had raced back away from the little one and was whirling around. Then he flew up the aisle in what looked like a single step, slammed his foot to the flagstone, and bellowed his first attack.

I strained like a horse on a fast rein. I put my mind ahead, into the war. And I did hear, at least a piece, and it was like the beginning of my life.

"... And sickness, and old age, and death! They have no cause! They cannot be stopped!"

The little monk stared up like a frightened rabbit and said some ancient words—the only part I caught was "Not t-t-t-true!"

The attacker let fly with a new stream of ideas that I couldn't understand at all. I clutched Grandmother's hand in frustration but I knew there was no help there. I would have to do it myself. I leaned forward and stared at the little monk's mouth, thinking it would help me hear if I could see his lips make the words. "The k-k-key!" he said. "In the mi-, mi-, the middle."

More spears thrown from the attacker. Ancient words. Nothing for me. And his dance was intensifying. As much as I disliked Drom I had to admire how he fought his war: leaping, singing, laughing, throwing his nets around his opponent. Every time a blow struck true—every time the little monk was struck without a ready reply—a cheer rang up from the rows of classmates looking on. I felt bad for the little monk—he obviously had a problem of some kind, a kind of a stutter, and as he grew more and more flustered it got worse and worse.

"Three p-p-p-poisons!" he cried.

"What three poisons, you s-s-simpleton!" taunted the big boy.

"The real c-c-causes of death! Real causes of getting... sick... or, or old! And how to, to st-st-stop them..." and then the little boy just couldn't go on, and he stared furiously at the ground.

But Tenzing flew to him, as I wanted to fly to him, and in that moment I saw that my brother was everything I had ever believed—graceful, handsome, and most of all, good—and I began to cry. Tenzing leaped up, and spun himself around, and sat down right next to the little monk, his arm around his shoulders. He thrust his other arm out at Drom with his beads clenched in his fist, as though he were about to unleash a bolt of lightning. I glanced quickly at Grandmother.

"The rules of the war," she rushed. "If a defender needs help, another may rise and join him. And anyone else can get up to add to the attack."

"The three poisons of the mind," cried out Tenzing bravely. "Represented by the three creatures, the key is in the middle of the Wheel of Life." And I understood every single word.

Drom paused in the middle of a whirl, and came down softly, like a cat, with glee in his eyes. "The real causes of old age?" he cried. "Three little animals, on a simple painting?"

"Just so!" and Tenzing threw the words back at him like boulders of iron.

"What really causes people to get sick? To get old? Even to die?" sang Drom, and began his dance again. He threw a look down into the rows of monks and two of them rose, as if on cue, to join him in the dance. I saw Stick, and then I saw Hammer. The two evil ministers of the mean little king.

"Just so!" shot back Tenzing, and the little monk in his arm looked up as well—timidly, but with some defiant fire of hope in his eyes.

Drom nodded at his friends and they flew forward in a line, stamping furiously before Tenzing and the rabbit. "The real causes of death? Of getting old? Of every disease there is? Causes that can be..." and they clapped their hands altogether at once, like thunder: "... stopped?"

"Just so!" roared back Tenzing, nearly lifted off his seat.

"Then why," said the terrible three, whirling as one in the air before my brother, "then why... do people still die?" And they threw their arms up in the air, exultant, swirling.

Tenzing gazed ahead, with a terrible look in his eyes, and it felt like a blade had been slipped into the middle of my chest, and all of a sudden, even before the others sitting there, I knew that he had no answer, and I suddenly looked down at the dark ground, because I could not bear to see what I somehow knew would come. And then there was a great cry of victory from all the monks with Drom, and the Debate Master was suddenly there, and he was waving his shawl again, and the groups of monks all over suddenly rose as one and began filing slowly out of the courtyard. And then it was all silent, and the clusters of old people were breaking up too and heading home, and a young monk was walking around the inside of the wall to collect the torches.

I turned to Grandmother. "Grandmother Tara—I need to know, I need to see the Wheel of Life. I need to see the three creatures. I need to know."

She glanced at me quickly, in the near dark, and nodded her head simply and quickly. "Come, come quickly," she pulled my hand.

9.

A Stranger in White

We walked quickly back along the wall, to the front and the gate to the courtyard. There was a jumble of people there, parents stopping their sons on the way back to their quarters in the monastery, to push a little bundle of sweets or fruit into their hands and say "You were wonderful!" Grandmother got held up for a moment by the tailor's wife from the village; I caught sight of Tenzing, working out through the crowd, still with an arm around the little monk's shoulder. I ran to them.

"Tenzing! Oh, it was so wonderful! It was so amazing!" I cried.

My brother looked at me ruefully, but this time it was the little monk who came to the rescue.

"W-w-well, we didn't do that well t-t-tonight, but you should have s-s-seen Tenzing doing the a-a-attacking, a f-f-few nights ago!" he beamed.

"My m-m-m-my!" came a loud voice behind him, along with a shove. The little monk whirled around, and suddenly the three of us were face to face with Drom and Stick and Hammer. "I think Di-di-la has got himself a little friend j-j-just his size!" roared Drom. Hammer leaned down towards me as if he were inspecting an ant, and then straightened up and blustered, "I think you're right, D-d-drom! And she talks just like him!"

"Why yes!" threw in Stick. "I recall her exact words—'Oh Uncle, I-I-I brought your t-t-tea!' Remember guys?" and they all three roared and pushed on past us.

Tenzing stared after them with a little scowl. "No wonder Uncle is always making him stay late after class. I bet he gets piles of extra work for all the trouble he makes."

But the little monk just slapped him on the back and said cheerfully, "Let it go, Tenzing. We'll get 'em next t-t-time. Now come up to my room for a few minutes, and we'll have some tea and plan our strategy for t-t-tomorrow."

Then he turned to me and said in a sincere voice, "And I'd be proud to be your friend, little sister. My name's Di-di-la," he joined his palms at his chest, in a Tibetan hello. "And what's your name?"

"They call me Friday," I smiled up at him— and then before he could ask me how come I had a boy's name I asked him, "Di-di-la; is that your real name?"

"Of course not," he smiled in return. "There's hardly a young monk in the whole monastery that gets called by his real name— everybody has a nickname, usually from some big embarrassing boo-boo they made at one time or another. But nobody takes it personally; I think mine's good luck even."

"But what does it mean?" I asked.

"Well you know there's that prayer to Gentle Voice, the Angel of Wisdom; the one that goes *om-a-ra-pa-tsa-na-di*, and you say it over and over on your beads, and on each bead first you take a big breath, and when you get to the *'di'* you say it as many times as you can, *di-di-di-di-di-di*, until you're completely out of breath, and then you go on to the next bead. And that's supposed to help you get smarter, and give you wisdom, so all the young monks say it a lot. And Drom, you know,

one day I was stuttering really bad at the beginning
of a debate, because I stutter when I get nervous,
and I couldn't even get past the *Di!* that you yell
first, and he laughed and said to everybody that it
sounded like I was saying that prayer, *di-di-di-di;*
and so I got stuck with it for a name."

"Does my brother have a nickname too?" I
suddenly thought to ask.

"Oh yes," said Di-di-la, with a twinkle in his
eye, "Of course! But that's something you better
ask him to tell you." I glanced up at Tenzing and
saw a look of relief.

Grandmother was still in the clutches of the
tailor's wife, some heavy gossip tonight, and I
decided to try to learn more.

"The beads—the string of beads you all wear
around your wrist." I pointed to the old worn
beads that Di-di-la wore, and then looked fondly at
the walnut rosary and turquoise mother-bead in
Tenzing's hands, something I remembered from
the first day I'd ever seen his dear face. "Why do
you wave them around when you fight? Does it
hurt when you get hit with them?"

Di-di-la laughed, his buck teeth opening into
a great wide smile. "Oh, no one ever hits anybody
in the courtyard wars. That's a very strict rule, and

it's lucky for me," he chuckled, "considering the size of Drom and his buddies. But you do wave your beads around and point them like you were pulling a bow back to shoot an arrow—it's all part of the game to try and distract your opponent. It teaches us to think clearly, even under pressure. If you can concentrate with that racket going on, you can concentrate anywhere, anytime. And the beads are also useful for remembering lists of stuff, like the twelve parts of the Wheel of Life," he concluded, still smiling at me, and eager to have me understand—just like Tenzing.

With this I remembered my questions, and looked again to Grandmother; Di-di-la seemed to sense that I needed to go and pulled Tenzing towards the nearest gate in the great wall around the monastery. "Get going, venerable one," he said, "or it will get so late I'll never be able to sneak you out the gates."

"Friday, tell Grandmother Tara I want to practice a bit with Di-di-la, okay?" asked Tenzing. "I'll be home right after that."

Tenzing was so honest and sincere that my grandmother and parents never doubted him, and neither did I. I gave him a nod and went and saved Grandmother from the rest of the village news.

"Oh, I forgot," she said, looking down at me, and then nodding to the tailor's wife. "We have something... rather important you know... to discuss with the Debate Master, the Vice-Abbot; with Geshe Lothar himself," she winked to her friend. "I'm sure you'll excuse us."

The other woman raised a significant eyebrow, and nodded back, and we turned and pushed in through the last of the young monks leaving the courtyard.

"People are allowed in after the debates let out," she smiled at me. She paused and looked towards the great pavilion. "Ah, there he is."

Grandmother put on her official look and towed me across to the pavilion, and up the stairs. Geshe Lothar was there, directing the last of the closing of the courtyard for the night.

"Vice-Abbot, eminent one," bowed Grandmother, formally. "Might we ask for a moment of your time?"

"Sure!" he boomed in reply—for as I came to learn, and love, he was never one for formality.

"My child, my granddaughter, Friday here, well... she wanted to ask a question, something about what the younger warriors were debating tonight."

Geshe Lothar looked down at me with a brief, intense gaze and then changed back again and swooped me up on the bench there, so I was nearly as tall as him. "Go ahead, my little Geshe," he laughed. "I'll do the best I can!"

"The Wheel," I said, gathering courage in the sunlight of his jolliness. "The Wheel of Life— what does it look like? How does it work? Is it true that there are three animals, and that they are what make people get sick or old or die?"

Geshe Lothar's eyes opened wide, and he turned and looked at Grandmother for a long, still moment. Then he gazed back into my eyes.

"Why turn around, child, and see for yourself," he said softly.

I turned, and there before me was one of the great pillars that hold up the center, the very highest part of the pavilion roof. And something was painted on it.

There was a monster, a big one, with huge angry eyes and fangs. And he had great strong arms and hands with long sharp claws. And in his claws he grasped a wheel, and deep inside the wheel there were three terrible creatures: a wild boar, and a snake with an evil glare, and a preening dove. The tail of the snake, and the tail of the dove, were snared tightly in the jaws of the boar. And then there were little worlds all around them, some filled with people, some with all the animals there are, and others with sad starving spirits and people burning and crying, and my heart cried out to them, and then I couldn't look any more and I turned my face and my tears back to Geshe Lothar.

"But what does it mean?" I whispered.

"Oh, there is so much to tell you," he whispered back to me, his eyes glistening. And then there was a young monk at his side, the one who had been taking down the torches from the wall, and he was pulling urgently on the Debate Master's shawl.

"Venered One, Elder," he said breathlessly. "Something you should see, something in the back." He gestured with his hand toward the back of the courtyard, close to where Tenzing's class had battled this night.

"What's that?" said Geshe Lothar, squinting into the darkness. "What's the matter? Show me."

The young monk pulled him along, and they stepped down from the pavilion to the flagstones, walking quickly. Grandmother's ears went up, and she grabbed me by the hand and helped me off the bench and marched off behind the two monks, as though official business were always her business, which it was.

I noticed then that there were still some warriors left in the courtyard, in little clusters here and there, near a lonely torch or two—they were talking excitedly, and occasionally broke out into dances and claps. "The hard-core," said Grandmother to me quietly, as we walked along. "The ones who really want to know. They were probably in the middle of a really good idea when the Debate Master went around and called off the battles for the night. Everyone else runs home to have tea; the ones who really need to know stay, until they know; sometimes it goes on until the dawn comes." She glanced around with a look of pride, as if they were all her warriors.

Then suddenly Geshe Lothar and the young monk pulled up short in the darkness of some shadows near the side wall; Grandmother and I came up silently at their sides.

"Over there, Elder One," said the young one. "Out in the fields, behind the torch at the back." I looked up and saw three or four young monks in a huddle, hurling questions and holy ideas at each other, in the light of a single torch on the wall

106

behind them. And then out beyond the torch, in the dark of the night, was the man.

He was not young; in fact, I think, he was old, but that was only in his face and his eyes. He had a strong face and a strong slender body, like my brother Tenzing. The night had already turned cold but he stood calmly with only a light, white cotton cloth wrapped around his waist, and another draped lightly over his bare chest. There was a thin white cord that went from his left shoulder down to his waist on the right, and then back around.

Leaning up against his shoulder was a staff of very old, worn wood—it was long, as tall as he was. The man was gazing at the monks intently, his eyes burning brightly with interest, brighter than the torchlight that filled his face. He was oblivious to our presence, as the young monks were to his. All we could do was look silently in a kind of awe at the fire in him, for a few minutes, and then finally the young monk broke the silence.

"A thread sage, Elder One!" he hissed.

"Ah, yes," returned Geshe Lothar, calmly. "That I can see."

"He's been standing there, listening, for quite some time, Revered One," gasped the novice.

"Really?" replied Geshe Lothar.

"Probably, you know, like they say, probably hoping to steal what we know," declared the younger man.

"Could be," said Geshe Lothar obligingly. "Or maybe," he said firmly, turning to the other full in the face, "maybe he just wants to know."

And then the younger monk's eyes dropped to the ground, flustered, and there was a long uncomfortable silence, and I looked at the strange man in white and suddenly my heart went out to him, because I suddenly realized that he was just like me—he was standing out there in the darkness, on the other side of the wall; he really wanted to come into the courtyard, and join in the goodness that was going on there, and he really wanted to know, he really needed to know, and maybe even there was someone who needed help and he wanted to help them and he knew that what he needed to help them was there in the courtyard somewhere—but for some reason he couldn't come in, they wouldn't let him in, there was something wrong with him, like there was something wrong with me, and why won't they let us in?

I pulled on Geshe Lothar's sleeve. I had to know. He turned and looked down at me, and then paused, and looked back at the man in white, but he was already gone.

Geshe Lothar sighed and looked at Grandmother. "Perhaps another time," he said kindly. "It is getting late, and the gates will be closing."

Grandmother nodded and said tersely, "Of course, Venerable One. She bowed, and we turned, and I left all my questions there. Except one.

We were walking back home in the familiar darkness of the horse road. Grandmother had opened the little red pouch that she always carried in her belt, and popped a little square of dried cheese in my mouth to suck on. But it didn't work so well, because I had learned how to push it into my cheek and keep on asking my questions. And so after a while I said, "Grandmother Tara, who was that man? And what is a thread sage?"

We kept walking and Grandmother gazed up at the stars before us and said quietly, "Oh, I don't really know a lot about it," and she paused, as I wondered on this odd admission. "You know, little Friday, I didn't grow up in this country." Then she stopped and looked down at me thoughtfully. "But you know, sometimes a person from another country can see things going on in a place that the people who live there don't see, because they're so close to it, you see."

Then she led me ahead for a spell and said, "The thread sages—they are like monks really, they have decided to devote their whole lives to helping people, in an ultimate way. But they don't live in monasteries; they live alone in some place that's quiet and far away from things—say in a forest, or in a cave. Or else they just wander alone from place to place, and accept whatever place to sleep or thing to eat that some kind person might offer to them. And they have a special knowledge—they know how to help people, to fix people, through special ways of moving your body, or even just breathing, and some special prayers and meditations that the monks maybe don't know much about.

"And the monks, you see, they too have special ways of helping people, of fixing people; but they go at it more through the mind, through understanding, and their own special prayers and meditations.

"And you see, whenever there are two groups like that—well, you know, there can be some people in both groups who are not so smart, and so they get jealous maybe of the people in the other group, especially when they can do something special, and then these little-minded people, you see, they talk a lot and stir up trouble between the two groups. And so a sad thing has happened now, and the monks and the thread sages stay pretty much away from each other, and there has even been some serious trouble..." she paused, and then seemed to decide it would not be good for me to hear.

"Which is all a very sad thing," she sighed, looking up again towards the stars over the road ahead of us. "Because, you see, in the old days, back in India, long ago, the monks also practiced the arts of the thread sages, and the thread sages followed the ways of the monks, and anyone who was seriously living as one was living as the other. And they say that someone who knew both could do a special healing; they could heal all sickness, and all sadness, in themselves—and they spent their lives showing others how to do it. Some even say," she paused there, in the middle of the road, "that they learned how to meet angels, the people of the sky..." she looked up again, "... and, and went to be with them, and learned to be angels themselves." We walked.

"It sounds so wonderful, Grandmother Tara," I mused. "Then why don't the people who understand, I mean, the grownup people, like you Grandmother, why don't they just go and get some good monks like Uncle and some thread sages like that man we saw tonight, and sit down all together, like in a big, big yurt somewhere, and get the monks to show the sages the part they know and get the sages to show the monks the part they know, and then everyone can fix themselves and go out and show other people how to fix themselves?"

Grandmother just kept walking and gazing up at the stars, and I looked at her face in their faint light—it had some strange soft mix of longing and sadness in it. "Oh, I don't know, little Friday," she said quietly.

"Then what about you?" I insisted, stopping us abruptly in the road. "What about just you, Grandmother? If the monks know something, if they really understand that Wheel of Life, and if they really know how to stop people from getting sick or old—if they even know how to stop people, people like Grandfather say, from dying—or if they only know a part, and maybe a thread sage could teach you the other part you need, then why, why Grandmother, why don't you go to them and ask to learn it?"

This time Grandmother's face came down to mine almost with a look of anguish, and also something I had never seen there before—it was uncertainty.

"Oh I don't know why, little Friday. It's hard in this country, you know, to do these things, if you're a woman..." Something touched me and I jerked and squeezed her hand, hard. She smiled then and continued, "... not that I would let that stop me.

"No, no, if I am really honest, it is not that," she sighed. "It is that I am really, inside, like just about everybody else. I get up in the morning and there's work to be done to make the tea or the bread, and then later on I get busy, and I'm thinking about family things or I go out and meet some friends from the village, and we talk, and I go home and eat, and then I'm tired out and ready for sleep; and, and well, life just flows on and takes me with it, and it lulls me like warm water, and then one day you wake up and you're old you see, old like me, and you feel like you're too old, and it's too late, and it just feels easier not to try to learn those things."

"But... I mean... even if you could learn how to save someone's life? To show them how to save their life themselves?"

She looked down at me sadly. "Oh, I don't know little Friday. It's so hard to change, and it's so hard to believe. You are so lucky to believe. You must try to keep that..." And she pulled me along, gently.

Knowing what could be, only just maybe, but that maybe being more important than everything else there was, I still couldn't understand why Grandmother didn't do something. I wanted to ask her more but I just kept it inside and walked quietly for a bit.

We were just coming up to the family yurt, and I could smell the smoke of the home fire in the cold sky, and I remembered one more thing.

"Grandmother Tara?"

"Yes," she said, sounding very tired, not like herself at all.

"Grandmother, the thread sages—why do they call them that?"

"Well because they wear this special cord, like the one you saw on the man tonight, the one that goes around their shoulder and then down like that.."

"But what does it mean?" I demanded.

"To tell you the truth, I'm not sure," laughed Grandmother. "But someone once told me that the cord represents the knowledge, the special knowledge of healing, that stretches down like a thread—from a teacher to a student, and from the student to their student—for hundreds and hundreds of generations. So when they feel the thread on their body, or they look down and see it, then it reminds them of their own Teacher, and of their Teacher's teachers, and of how kind those people are to teach what they know, and pass it on, and keep it alive in the world.

"And as you can see, they don't wear a whole lot else!" she laughed again.

"But why not?" I asked again, trying to hold her there but feeling suddenly very sleepy myself.

"Oh, you see, they do these special kind of movements—like exercises, you see—and special kinds of breathing, and praying, and such, and they say it begins to change your body, and then if you do it right your body just all changes, and well— that's what they say at least—you know, like I said, you sort of just change into an angel, and your body then is made of light.

"But even before you get that far, they say, you know—I'm not really so sure about how it all works and so on—you just start to feel so good and strong inside that you're warm as a steamed bun, all the time, no matter what the weather. Why, I've even heard that the thread sages who are women don't wear anything more than that man you saw tonight, when they do their special exercises, because they have to learn to make the warmth come from the inside, not the outside—it's like, you see, some kind of first step I think, and then I heard too…" but then Grandmother stopped abruptly, and peered down at me with a nervous look.

"Thread sages… who are women?" I said, staring up at her intently.

"Why yes," she said, slowly, I think wondering how to take the words back. "But there's very few of them. In fact, I think you could say not a single one maybe in this whole part of the country!" she added perkily.

But the damage was done, and we both knew it, and she sighed heavily. "Come girl," she put her arm around me. "Time to get some sleep. You can't do everything in one day." She pulled me along into the warmth of the family fire, and the family.

10.

Needles

Over a year went by like that—I was growing up fast, Grandmother was growing old fast, and we went as often as I could get her to go, to see the warriors of wisdom battle. In a good week we might go three times, cutting through the back way, over the slate ridge, to save time sometimes on the way out—although it was too dangerous to come back that way, in the dark. On the other days I kept my vigil at the stone shrine, with Tara—the Lady of Freedom—and sang silently with Tenzing.

I could recognize a good part of these songs in the debates that the warriors waged, but Uncle was pushing them on hard, and without hearing his classes I knew I would never grasp it at all. They had moved on from the Wheel of Life to new things within a month or two—walking by Uncle's yurt during the day I could catch tantalizing bits, but only when they were practicing the warriors' special claps and cries: Uncle would pretend to be an attacker and yell an idea out at the top of his lungs, and then all the boys were expected to yell the answer back and clap on time.

I began to notice that there were certain rules to the answers—it seemed like they could only be one of four or five short phrases—but they were all old words, close to the Mother Tongue, and I could only guess at their meaning. And so really I was always only straining from the other side of a wall, whether it was the stone wall of the warrior's courtyard or the felt-covered wall of Uncle's yurt.

It was the autumn of that year when everything began to change. It started really when Tenzing, who was growing stronger and taller and more handsome with every passing month, ran to me breathless one morning after class.

"Oh Friday! Guess what! Uncle says we've finally finished with Perfection of Wisdom, and next week we get to do the Old Man!"

Whenever Tenzing got excited I got excited too, even if I didn't know anything about whatever was exciting him. Later on I learned that the Perfection of Wisdom was the first of the Five Great Books that a young monk had to master on the way to becoming a Geshe. Finishing it was a big step for the boys—a step that in some monasteries might take seven years. But I was only seven myself at the time and didn't know about all those things. It was the Old Man part that sounded interesting.

"What's the Old Man, Tenzing?" I bubbled, grabbing his hand.

"Oh, it's really wonderful. You wouldn't believe it. You see, to celebrate finishing the First Book, we get to march around the monastery dressed up in these amazing costumes. The Old Man I guess is some kind of king from the old days. And he has his right-hand man, his Prime Minister. And then there's a couple of big tough bodyguards, who lead them around, and also a kind of goofball who's the Court Jester, or whatever.

"So we tramp around the monastery for the whole morning, and the bodyguards make lots of noise and yell 'Ho! Here comes the Old Man! Make way there!' and everybody has to move out of the way. And then every once in a while we can stop, anywhere we like in the whole monastery, and everybody crowds around, and then the Old Man you see he points to somebody in the crowd, could be anybody, you see, and then the Prime Minister nods to one of the bodyguards, and he steps up to that person—no matter who it is, really—and waves his big fake sword at him and yells, 'You there! Step up to the Old Man! You are ordered to answer his questions!'

"And they pull the guy up to the Old Man and he asks them some very silly questions, and no matter who it is—I'm talking about even people like Uncle, or the Precious One himself, the Abbot!—well they have to come and pay their respects to the Old Man, and answer any funny question he asks them!

"So you see—get this—Uncle himself could be walking down the road, and the Old Man could call him over, and say, 'Hey you there! I think I know you! Aren't you that teacher who always gives the young monks way too much homework to do? And oh, by the way—do you have any good explanation for just why all your classes last week were so *boring?'* And then Uncle or the Abbot or whoever it is has to play along and give a good answer and the whole crowd ends up roaring with laughter!"

He laughed too and I laughed and pulled on his hand with excitement. A chance to grill the know-it-all adults! A chance to turn the tables on them! Let them figure it out when we say things that don't make any sense! But then I thought of something else, and my face fell.

"But can anybody come and watch, Tenzing? Anybody who wants to?"

"Anybody!" he bellowed. "No! *Everybody!* It's the most fun of the whole year! You'd be crazy to miss it!"

Then one more thing occurred to me. "And you, Tenzing—do you get to be somebody important?" I asked adoringly.

He broke into a huge smile and said, "Well, you know, Drom and Hammer are so big and tough, well they were naturals to get picked as the Old Man's bodyguards. Stick is tall and never smiles and is all shrewd like, so he of course got chosen as the Prime Minister. Di-di-la with his big funny eyes and buck teeth and that stutter he's got, and well, just because he's a fun guy all the time anyway, he's got to be the Court Jester.

"So that left me to be..." he began.

"The Old Man himself!" I squealed with joy, and then we threw our hands up and started laughing and dancing in a big circle around the clearing, until finally Uncle had to poke his head out and shush us—but not without a big smile too.

The night before the big day Tenzing and I were too excited to sleep. We laid there on a little

pile of new carpets that Amala had woven, with
our heads up close to the family fire, because it was
already quite cold, and would stay that way until
the sun was well up in the sky. I was thinking hard,
about really embarrassing questions that I could
suggest to Tenzing to ask the adults. There were
three butter lamps for good luck going all night on
the altar across the fire pit from us, throwing a
cheerful golden light around the yurt. They
seemed a reflection of my own heart—our family
was so happy, so many good things were
happening, I had such a wonderful strong brother
and clever good parents and a grandmother who
was my best playmate but my steadfast shelter at
the same time. And so I thought dreamily for quite
a while, until we could hear Father's snores on one
side, and Grandmother's fidgety sleep on the other
side. Then Tenzing poked me in the ribs and we
put our heads close together and had our night-
time talk—all stifled giggles and strategies for
confusing the adults; I remember one last question
about whether the Old Man could also put his
bodyguards on the spot—it seemed a perfect
opportunity to get back at Drom and Hammer—
but Tenzing said he didn't think so, and then Father
was crouching down next to us in the cold and
gently shaking us awake.

He and Amala were already dressed up in
their fine silk greatcoats, with the bright sashes
around the waist. They looked so nice to wake up

to. Grandmother was still up in her fancy little bed amidst the carved chests and tables; she was laying there on her side, with her head up on one elbow and her long beautiful gray hair flowing down all around the pillows, surveying her domain with a sleepy, regal look.

"You two run along now, with Tenzing," she yawned. "I'll come after a bit with little Friday. No way I'm sitting through a couple of hours of prayers in a big cold temple while they all get blessed for the next book they have to study. We'll be there outside when it's time for the Old Man to appear," and she winked at Tenzing and me, and drew the quilts and her old furs back up around her shoulders.

There was a little tussle while Amala pulled out some nice and warm but very scratchy new woolen robes for Tenzing, who refused to change out of his comfortable worn-out cotton ones, until Father made one of his usual deals and agreed to let Tenzing walk the whole way with the Old Man's long white beard hanging off his belt. It was a really wonderful beard and came down all the way to Tenzing's waist; Father had fashioned it cleverly from a good number of long fine hairs snipped from the tail of Snow-White, one of his favorite caravan yaks.

I was too excited to lie back down again, so I went out to say goodbye. Uncle appeared too, his sad brown eyes bright as always in the early morning—he never seemed sleepy then.

"Well congratulations again," he smiled to Tenzing, patting him heartily on the back. "Keep a good heart during the prayers; and best of luck with that... er... Old Man thing!"

Tenzing and I both jolted and stared at him at the same time. "But Uncle," I protested. "Does that mean you're not coming to watch?"

"Uh... er... lots of stuff to do here," he spluttered, but we knew he had the day off and was probably just looking forward to spending it shut up in his room with some of his books. This was how many of the senior teachers, it turned out, spent the Old Man's day as well.

"And anyway," added Uncle, "someone's got to watch the homestead!" He gave a serious nod to Father, who just rolled his eyes with a smile and pulled Tenzing and Amala along. They took to the horse road, where lots of villagers and their sons would be up and headed for the prayers. It wasn't Amala's way to talk a lot with other people as they walked, but she did know that everyone would see from the beard that "her little Geshe" was going to play the starring role.

Grandmother was especially slow getting up; I dragged in one of the wooden buckets of water from outside and set it next to the family fire, so the ice would melt off the top. Then I added some logs to the fire, trying to induce Grandmother to come out from under the covers. I wasn't allowed to make the morning tea yet—I was still too small to even reach the top of the tea churn, much less work the plunger—but I filled the big kettle and set it next to the fire to warm. Then all I could do was sit down and wait anxiously for Grandmother. Oftentimes in the morning I would sing to myself, in my own mind, parts from the holy books I'd learned, for practice. But it didn't come when I was thinking too much about something else, like the Old Man.

It seemed like hours later—but it was still dark—when Grandmother finally sat up. She looked tired and grumpy while she brewed the tea, setting some aside in a small churn for Uncle to come get later. Then she made her morning offering of juniper smoke to the sky gods of her native land; it seemed very quiet that time, and her mind was gone with them for a long while. Then she sat on the side of her bed and began to poke around with a distracted look, trying to find something.

"What is it, Grandmother?" I asked, a little worried that we might be late.

"*Kaprel,*" she muttered. "Can't seem to find the *kaprel.*"

The *kaprel* was one of Grandmother's most prized possessions—it was a little metal tube with a lid that held all her sewing needles. Needles were a rare commodity in our day—the coarse, local ones were made by spending hours and hours filing down a lump of iron. The better ones—and Grandmother had a good collection of these—were from India, far to the south. They had to be brought in by caravan, a long and dangerous journey over the snow mountains; but after all this was Father's business.

"*Kaprel,* for what?" I cried.

"Oh, ah..." she murmured, still looking around under all her things. "Got to sew something—got to finish sewing something."

I groaned inside. We were sure to be late, on the most important day of all—the day that Tenzing and I would have our fun on the grown-ups. "Finish what?" I wailed.

"Oh, that lovely piece of silk, the one from India, that your father gave me last week. Said I could make it into a blouse to wear today, special. Your father is so wonderful that way, almost as sharp as your grandfather was!" she proclaimed to the ceiling, and then began to rummage around again.

"But we have to get going," I whined. "We'll be late! We might miss some of the Old Man! Why didn't you finish it before?"

"Because I... I..." she mumbled, still sleepy or something, I couldn't tell. "Oh!" she exclaimed, and stopped frittering around, and snapped up straight. "I couldn't finish it because I was sewing something else, all week, in secret!" she suddenly recalled. And then Grandmother reached behind her pillow and pulled out a little package wrapped in a gaily colored cotton cloth. She handed it to me, with a soft, sort of confused smile.

I unwrapped the cloth, and there inside first I saw a lovely piece of sky-blue silk. I pulled it out and saw it was a beautiful new blouse, made my size. I've never been one to worry much about clothes, but it was really quite fine, and I gave a big smile and reached up onto the bed and hugged Grandmother around the waist. She smiled happily and poked at the cloth. "Look, there's more," she chuckled.

And then I saw there was a new woolen *chuba* there—a sort of grayish blue, just my size too. A *chuba* is a kind of dress that Tibetan ladies almost always used to wear. It has a long nice skirt that goes all the way down to your ankles. Attached to that is a top piece that goes up all the way in the back and about halfway up in the front, and you button them together at your shoulder. Then the blouse goes underneath and shows in the front and at the collar and sleeves, really pretty. Grandmother made me put them on and go stand over in the firelight so she could see.

"Oh that's perfect," she said dreamily. "You look all pretty blue, like the sky, as if one of the sky angels had come down, just for today.

"I only did the blouse," she added. "Getting hard for me to see almost anything, much less sew. The tailor's wife did the rest; a pretty fair job I'd say," and she patted down some seams.

"Now where did the *kaprel* go to?" she suddenly recollected herself, and began nervously picking around at her things again. "It's not a lot, just got to add some brocade to the sleeves," and she held up her new blouse.

It was the same as mine; I giggled to think of how she had wheedled a piece out of Father big enough for both of us, and Grandmother smiled back at me gently.

Then she dug around through all her piles of things again; after a while the newness of the dress wore off, and I was up on the bed, more and more frantic, helping her open little boxes and bags. I looked down at her blouse.

"But Grandmother, you know, it's already such a lovely blouse. I don't think you need to add a thing to it," I said, really afraid we were going to miss the Old Man altogether. "And I think maybe it's, well, getting late."

She raised her face close to mine and some of that steel look came back in her eyes and she said, "No, little Friday. It's got to be just right.

"It's things," she went on, "the things you have." And she waved her arms all around her, to the little piles of possessions she had accumulated over the course of all those years. "They should be nice. Things should be *nice*. People should have *nice things*," and she stared at me hard through the bleary eyes, as if struggling to convince herself of something. Then her face softened and she shifted to her Authority-of-the-Family voice.

"And don't you worry, little Friday," she said, patting my hand. "We'll be right on time. I have it all planned out. We'll take the shortcut over the ridge—it will be getting light by then—and then we'll walk back home on the horse road, and it will be broad daylight, and everyone will be able to see our new outfits." Then to cement the deal she reached over to the little red pouch on a chest at the side of her bed, and shook out a cheese square for me to chew on, to keep me quiet. And out popped the *kaprel*.

"Oh!" exclaimed Grandmother simply. "I knew I put it somewhere where you and I'd find it!" And she gave me the cheese and picked up the *kaprel* and pulled off the top with her hands shaking and all the needles spilled out in a jumble, falling to the floor, sharp little points on the cold stone.

Everything began to seem strange then. I am down in the dark under the bed, trying to find the needles, and they are sticking into my little fingers. Then Grandmother is muttering and trying to sew on the fancy cuffs, but they come out crooked—and the strangest thing, she doesn't even notice. And then we are walking out the back way, out the little path between the stone shrine and the cattle pen.

"Shouldn't we say goodbye to Uncle?" I ask.

"Oh no," she says in a distracted voice. She is looking up at the ridge ahead of us, or maybe at the sky above it. "He'll already be inside a book somewhere, or in some meditation. He probably thinks we left a long time ago, by the horse road."

And then she is pulling me along on the little row of dirt between the fields, "Don't step on the grain, dear," as if I didn't know every single stalk is precious. And her hand is ice cold and the wind is blowing hard against our backs and the sun is up but not out because thick gray clouds are covering that whole half of the sky. And all I can see is Grandmother's back and the blue silk and the brocade cuffs and the tall sheaves of winter wheat all around us.

And then after half an hour of hard walking we break out into the clearing, past the wheat, where the big pool is, and the ground is all frozen and hard and covered with holes left by the hooves of the cattle. And we turn downstream, to the right, like we always do, to cross the stream at the logs and rocks that make the dam for the pool.

And her cold hand, so cold, is still shaking, and she pulls me across the log we have crossed a thousand times, but this time at the end her foot slips a bit, and plunges into the icy water, but she gets that hard look of her face and says "Don't mind it, child," and pulls me now in some kind of hurry upstream on the other side, up past the pool. And we are up close to the ridge then, and she looks up at the top of it again—or at the sky? And by sheer willpower she pushes her old body up the hard-packed earth of the ridge path.

And then we are at the top, and we pause, and Grandmother is breathing very hard, and the tips of her cold fingers are pricking my little palms like the fallen needles. And the sun is still helpless behind the gray, behind us, and home is back far down there across the fields, the yurts as small as mushrooms.

And now down the far side, nearly dark, along the path that cuts steep across the ridge of cold gray slate. "Step carefully, little one. Not the place to fall, here," and she nods at the steep stone slope below us, and the cliff at the end, where the villagers and the monks have dug out half the hill for slates to make roofs and courtyard tiles.

And then we are picking our way carefully over sharp slippery plates of stone and she pulls up all of a sudden and raises that princess head tall and proud and stares hard down at some pines at the bottom and points her arm out like some stern goddess and says "Look at him!"

And I look hard but I can't see much in the gloom but then there's a movement down between the pines. And first I see the horns, like long curved swords, each longer than a man's leg. And then I see the mighty head, and finally the body, shoulders ten feet above the ground. And he is some great beast like a wild yak and he stops there halfway out the trees, and turns his terrible face up to us, and stares once, long and slow.

And then he is charging up the ridge, his shaggy head thrown back, jaws open, but no roar, silent, only the howl of breath in his throat. He covers the steep slope in leaps twenty feet at a time, haunches rippling, knife-sharp hooves digging into stone itself. Sheets of gray rock fly down and off the cliff, shattering at the bottom. The ridge itself quakes under our feet. And before we can take a single step he is upon us, huge, slavering, towering over our heads, bloody red eyes that rake across mine, first, and I feel the cold of hell, just there. And the eyes go over my shoulder and stop there on Grandmother, and they stay there, and nothing moves at all.

And then he just turned, quietly, gently, and trotted like a pony up the path that Grandmother and I had just come down. He reached the top of the ridge and walked out on a huge flat stone against the sky. He turned and looked back at us, looked the third time, the wind ripping into his hair, whipping it across the sky like a great battle flag. This time he didn't look at me. He only looked over me, behind me, to Grandmother.

And she gave a little cry, "Oh," and I will never forget it as long as I live. And I turned halfway around to see her and her face was lifted up towards his, or to the sky itself, and she was staring up hard, and her arms were all wrong, they were thrown out straight to the sides as if she were dancing before Father's fire.

And I turned and looked back up at the beast but he was gone, and the wind tore again, at the gray clouds, and they were great beasts themselves, at war, rending and tearing each other, and then they parted, in an instant, and there was a great chasm of pure blue sky, and the golden sun flooding free across it.

She stamped her feet, three times, in a rhythm, and my heart leaped, hoping it was just a dance, and I whirled around and she was there in the shaft of golden light and her head was thrown back to the sky and she made three graceful spins nearly into the air—

And then Grandmother pitched forward hard to the ground and began rolling down the stone, towards the edge of the cliff.

11.

Grandmother Just Get Up

The world went silent then—it was the first time it ever came on me, the silence. I was in my true element, for the first time, in a way that I would be for years at a time later in my life. A human life was thrown into my hands—to save, or to lose.

I leaped towards Grandmother to grab her arm but she rolled past and was gone. I fell and threw myself ahead on all fours, shards of the gray slate slashing my hands and ripping at my knees through the new wool. I grasped for her other hand as she rolled again but it was already gone; I made one last hopeless dive towards her and the silly long sleeve flew past and slapped me in the face and I closed my hand on it. It stretched and began to tear but it held—and it saved her dear life.

Grandmother stopped rolling, just for an instant, and in the still of the moment I threw myself forward, across her body. We slid a few feet more and came to a stop, not far from the cliff. I worked myself over her the rest of the way, and dug my toes into the slope, and held us both. I looked down into her face.

Her eyelids fluttered and she opened her eyes and looked up at my face and then past it, to the sky. Her features were soft and relaxed, almost in a smile, and it occurred to me that it was all some terrible joke.

"Oh Grandmother," I spoke to her softly, "oh, it's not funny. It's not funny. Come now and get up. And we'll go."

She just stared up past me, to the sky. I tried to pull her shoulder up and we slipped a few inches more and I said to her, louder now, "Come on, please. Just get up. Just get up, Grandmother."

And I stared at her eyes but they weren't moving at all, just fixed upon the sky. And then a fear began to gnaw in me, in my chest, deep inside, and I cried, "Grandmother! Grandmother Tara! Just get up!"

But she only closed her eyes softly and a gust of freezing wind burst across the rock and the pain from the cuts in my hands and my knees came to me in a shock and I wailed, "Just get up!" to no one at all, and from somewhere inside me the wind tore away all the warmth and safety of my life and left me afraid, very afraid, and the one who could help me was in my arms, nothing more than a child herself now, and something I had always known but was always afraid to think poured unleashed into my mind: that Grandmother, my Grandmother, and all the other grown-ups too, were just as weak and helpless and unknowing in this cold world as the smallest little child in their care. And it brought a sadness and a knowledge upon me that never really left again, and all I could do was lay my head down, lay it down in the cold wind, upon the frail warmth that remained in the old woman below me. And I sobbed, and she was still, for the longest time.

12.

Ripples in a Pool

Grandmother's body suddenly shuddered beneath mine, and it woke me from myself. I raised my head—the wind was gone for a moment—and tried to look over my shoulder to see how far from the cliff we were. Then she jolted, violently, and my feet, frozen from the cold, gave out. We were sliding across the face of the rock again.

A stone came up and hit Grandmother hard across the head, and I didn't even think, I just threw an arm across to try to protect her face and then my hand struck something coming up out of the rock, and I grabbed and held with all my might. It was the trunk of a little juniper, struggling out of a crevice in the stone. We stopped again, and the silence came on me again, and the doubts were gone, and I knew it was I who had to do something.

I got my shoulder behind the blessed little tree and then pulled Grandmother across to me, letting her slide a bit more but towards the tree. Then I struggled and got her across in front of me and wedged her little waist between the trunk and the angle of the slope. And then I bent over her again, calmly this time, and tried to make my voice strong and steady, like hers.

"Now Grandmother Tara, there's nothing to worry about. I've got you all tucked in here safely, and now I'm going to go up there to the top of the ridge and call down towards home, and get someone to come help us. I'll always be in sight and I'll keep looking down here too, to make sure you're all right. Do you understand me, Grandmother?" Inside I was ready to break down again, and it was so scary and wrong, talking this way to the one who should be talking to me this way. But she didn't say anything, anything at all. She looked up still with her eyes wide open, but now very, very sad eyes—glistening in the cold, as if she wanted to cry but there was something wrong and she couldn't even get the tears to leave her eyes. And so I just said "All right, then," and I tightened my dress up as well as I could and crawled away from her and up the steep cold rock.

It wasn't as hard with just myself, and I soon made the path. I turned around there to check on Grandmother but she was just still, still there, limp as a doll, staring at the sky with her jaw dropped open. And now I could see that we had stopped only a few feet from the edge of the cliff. I shivered and turned resolutely and worked my way straight up to the ridgetop.

The ground I had to cover was all boulders, with little tiny spaces between them jammed with junipers that tore at my clothes and my arms as I tried to squeeze through. In some places I had to climb up and over the great stones, balancing against the wind, and in other places I got down on my belly and squirmed through little holes between them, praying it was still too cold for the poison snakes to be out. And then finally I was almost to the top, at the base of one last great boulder that was wedged between two spires of stone rising another thirty feet into the air. I clambered up on my stomach again, pushing with my feet and my knees and prying my fingers into little cracks to pull myself up. And then I was up, and I could see home, down on the other side.

I got up on my knees and almost fell forward, slipping on the remains of an eagle's lair. Ahead was a sheer drop of hundreds of feet, almost straight down, to the big pool and the head of the path up the ridge. I squeezed the stone with my knees and put my hands down to balance and took another look over my shoulder, down at Grandmother. She was even smaller now, far away, still as death. I turned my head towards home and cried for help, with all the strength I could gather.

As if in answer a cold torrent of wind rushed up the ridge, funneled between the spires, and nearly threw me backwards off the peak. It tossed my little child's voice back in my face, cruelly, and flew off again to the sky. I burst out in tears. No one would ever hear me. I was cold and scared and I wasn't sure I could even get down to the path again.

Then once again it was silent, as if something or someone who lived between the gusts of wind were reaching out to help me; and it all got clear, and I knew what I had to do. I had to make the *zadak*, I had to make a loud noise that would slip right by the cruel wind and reach my home. I had to raise the alarm, the alarm that children were never—for any reason—allowed to raise.

I turned around and came straight down off the huge rock, without even thinking. I found two big flat stones that would fit in my tiny palms, and I got them and myself back up on the rock. And shaking like a leaf from the cold and the fear I smashed them together, to beat out the sound of the *zadak*, the alarm of deadly threat. One beat. A pause. Two beats, and then another pause, and scream *Zadak! Danger!* at the top of your lungs.

And the wind steals away the cry of the voice, but not the message of the stones.

I pounded and screamed and never stopped. I felt something wet in the coldness of my hands, and looked down and saw that one of my fingers had got caught between the stones and was bleeding badly—a little stream of crimson across the soft new blue silk of my blouse, puddling between the gashes torn through the new dress. But I didn't stop, and I stared down at home, willing someone to hear.

And then there was Uncle, striding around the edge of his yurt. He was too far away for me to see much of his face but I could see he was just pulling on his dark red monk's vest—I saw a flash of something white against his bare chest, and then he had tucked the vest shut. His head came up towards the top of the ridge, like an animal sniffing the air for danger. I knew I was too far away for his old eyes to see me, but I beat the stones with all my strength, and screamed to spite the wind.

And his head turned once to the left, towards the family yurt. Then again, to the right out past the cattle pens. And then in a single motion his arm flew to the side and caught up one end of his long red monk's shawl and cinched it up around his waist, and then he stepped towards the tall waving wheat and he just—he just changed.

And all I could see then was flashes of red blurring through the wheat—the wind would blow in a wave across the tops of the golden grain and lay them down in curling patterns, just for a second, and I would glimpse the loose end of Uncle's shawl trailing behind him, turning in sudden bursts like lightning, always into the wind—working into the strength of the wind, cutting into its power, using the wind by consuming the wind.

I could tell the flashes were heading towards the big pool. They covered the distance across the fields in less than a minute. I picked the spot where Uncle would break from the wheat and stared there, hard. I don't think I ever would have seen what I did if I hadn't.

The wheat burst open and Uncle was there frozen in half-stride. His face now was clear and it was up straight gazing ahead with the strangest look of calm, not a single wrinkle on it anywhere, no strain, as if he were deep asleep but the widest awake at the same time. The front of his shawl was plastered up against his chest from the sheer velocity, as though he were racing full out on a very fast horse.

I waited in that split second for him to turn downstream, to the log crossing, but he just came straight towards the big pool, without the slightest

143

hesitation. And then he suddenly was out of sight on this side, already coming up the ridge. I blinked and stared hard at the pool. There were four little circles across the face of the water, and even as I watched each of them began to send bigger circles of ripples out to the edge of the pool. I shook my head sharply and turned and got back down to the path as fast as I could, half running, half falling.

I stopped there where Grandmother and I had stood and seen the beast, and I looked at her down below so helpless and I started to cry again and suddenly there was Uncle at my side. He put his arm around my shoulders and hugged me hard, with that strange heat that always seemed to radiate from him. I pointed down to Grandmother and his eyes followed knowingly. Then he grasped my arm strongly in his hand and we made our way down to her.

Uncle made me take hold of the little juniper trunk with both hands, and then he let go of me and stooped down next to Grandmother. He took her hand gently in his own and rolled back the fancy little sleeve. And then he placed the tips of three of his fingers at some special spots around her wrist and closed his eyes and felt for something. He was quiet for a long time. Then his sad eyes opened up sadder than ever and he bent down slow whispering *atsi, atsi:* sadness, oh sadness. And something very cold came inside my chest, and I

144

knew that something was really terribly wrong with Grandmother, and I stared, helplessly, at the two helpless grown-ups.

13.

Going to the Well

Uncle turned and looked into my eyes and suddenly looked down—I don't know if it was something there he didn't want me to see, or something in me he couldn't bear to see.

Then he got up slowly and tightened his shawl around his waist with a knot and made me take hold of the end in both hands. He bent and lifted Grandmother in his arms, as easily as if she were a handful of cotton. And we started back home.

At the bottom of the ridge we came to the pool, and Uncle walked straight downstream to cross at the log. I stopped suddenly at the side of the stream, remembering something, and stared back at the pool for a moment. Uncle paused and turned and looked at me, just for a second. And then we had crossed the log and Uncle was marching straight for the family yurt—his sad burden in his arms and his eyes staring straight ahead—crushing a little trail through the golden grain.

I opened the door for Uncle and he stooped and we came in and he set Grandmother down there on her special bed, amidst all her things, her nice things. I looked at them and felt some kind of anger, I don't know why, as if the nice things had almost betrayed my Grandmother. They didn't seem nice at all. They were still there, but they were refusing to help the woman who had given them a home and cared for them so well, so long. I think it was then that I lost my trust in *things*.

We stood for a while, Uncle and I, at the side of her bed, just looking at Grandmother lying there. But she didn't look at us. Her eyes were wide open, like before, but she was already gone somewhere, already returned to a child, staring out the sky-window overhead as I had stared as a baby. And then the sadness and the cold and the cuts in my hands and legs all came down on me too hard and I burst out crying again, finally a little girl again, and Uncle stooped and took me in his arms and held me until I was quiet, and then in silence he washed and tended my wounds. And finally I could speak to him.

"Something very bad happened, Uncle," I began, very softly. "A creature came at us, a big,

big animal. And something happened with his eyes when he looked at Grandmother, and she fell down, and she began rolling down towards the cliff, and I jumped to stop her, and I fell, and we started sliding, and it was only that little tree..." And then I couldn't talk again for a while, but he was kind, and he didn't ask me anything, he just held me. I knew there was something else I had to say.

"And the *zadak*, Uncle," I started, slowly. "The *zadak*, the alarm, that you said children are never supposed to make, that it was a rule, and well I... I broke the rule."

"Oh little Friday," he smiled gently, his face right up to mine. "You did well. You did very well. Sometimes the best way to keep a little rule is to break it for something bigger." And I nodded, because I had felt that, and I knew he knew.

We were quiet for a moment more, and then I looked up into his sad gentle face again and said, "And Uncle, there is something... about what you did, there at the big pool..."

Suddenly I felt his strong hands tighten on my shoulder, and he frowned, and said, "So you did see that."

I nodded, and looked down, and Uncle was silent for a while. Then he lifted my chin in his hand and made me look him in the eye.

"Listen, little Friday. What you saw today was something very special... a special kind of, a kind of power. But nobody else should know about it. I want you to promise me you'll never tell anyone what you saw. Promise?" he said softly.

"I promise, Uncle." I said. And you should know I only tell you about it here because all those things were so long ago, and maybe it would help you to know.

Then he began to speak again. "And Friday, there's something... something you should know about it, about that power." Uncle paused.

"People, special people, can do things like what you saw, because they know where to go to get the power to do them," and he paused again, as though he were having trouble finding the right words.

"And the place that they go to, it's sort of like... like a well, where you go to pull up water. And there is power in the well, lots of power."

I just nodded. I felt like I understood.

He looked up a little uncertainly again and then back down at me. "But there's something very important about that power, and you need to know that. It is much more important than doing things like what you saw me do today."

I nodded again, and waited, for I felt the power of the moment, the power of special moments that only come to us a few times in our whole lives. And then he said, "The place where all the power comes from—the well that has deep inside it all the power really—is just plain kindness, just being kind to other people. The kind of kindness, the kind of power *you* showed today, when you jumped to help Grandmother, when you risked yourself to help someone else. That is the real power, because that is where all the other power comes from." And then he just stopped, and I could see he was afraid he hadn't said it clearly enough.

It was very clear though, very clear, and I needed to tell him—but he looked in my eyes one last time and saw it there, and he nodded, and he stood up. We stopped again, and stared sadly at Grandmother, staring too. Then something struck me, like a burst of light, and I turned to Uncle—a seven-year-old child to one of the greatest masters Tibet has ever seen—and I said, "I can fix her. I can fix Grandmother. I know what to do."

14.

How to Slay a Monster

Things were changing fast then. Amala got quieter and had to work even harder, or thought she did. Grandmother didn't seem to get any better, or any worse; she just laid there like a child, and Amala would feed her soup and clean up her messes. Uncle came in often the first few days and then less and less, as it became apparent there was not much to be done.

But I had a plan, and as soon as things settled down I went to Tenzing early in the morning one day and told him I was going to the big pool to wash up and play until lunch. Then on the way out I walked over close to Uncle's yurt— he was teaching a class and no one was looking— and I reached down and grabbed one of the big clay jugs that the milkmaid Bukla used when she came every morning to milk the cows. I hurried down to the big pool and put some water in the jug and then balanced it on my hip with my little arm around it, like I'd seen the women do. And then I clambered up over the ridge, keeping my eyes to the path—too hurt still to look where Grandmother had been—and made straight for the monastery, walking as fast as I could.

Women weren't generally allowed in the part of the monastery where the monks had their little rooms, but during the day this rule was relaxed if, say, a young girl from a family with cows had to deliver a jug of milk to a Lama for the day's tea.

I swept in through the main gates and headed over towards the monks' rooms as if I belonged there (one of the many things I'd learned from Grandmother Tara). I walked straight up to the first monk I saw who looked senior enough to ask me what I was doing there and declared, "Jug of milk for the Vice-Abbot, Geshe Lothar. Would you mind, Venerable One, to direct me to his quarters?" And he nodded hurriedly and turned around and walked quickly through some narrow alleyways between the little stone houses, cutting right across several porches with older monks out enjoying the sun. They looked at my guide and didn't give me a blink. In a few minutes I was afraid I would never be able to find my way out again.

Then in wonder I began to notice that I could hear classes, just like Uncle's, going on all around me, the holy words and the questions and the answers shouted back and the handclaps pouring out from window after window. I began to wish I *could* get lost there, and stay.

We crossed one last courtyard of gray slate from the ridge, and the old monk pointed to a steep flight of steps and said, "Right up there, second floor; can't miss it." And then he hurried off to wherever he'd been going in the first place.

I struggled up the stairway, two flights really, one doubled back over the other, with the jug of water—which by now had become very heavy, even half full.

At the top, on a broad landing under an overhang, was a low, sturdy wooden table, with some old rugs thrown on the ground around it. I saw Geshe Lothar sitting there on one of the rugs, with two gentle-looking young novices at his side. He turned and greeted me with a huge smile; the sunlight angled in and lit up his jolly features, and I felt like everything would be all right.

"Uh, Geshe Lothar, Vice-Abbot, sir, respected one, I, uh..." I began ingraciously, and then just pointed suggestively at the pot cradled in my elbow.

He paused only for a blink and then boomed, "Ah! The milk! Excellent!" Then he turned to the older of the two boys and said very seriously, "Lunrik! I say! Did the stairs have a sweep today?"

"Why yes, Elder One," he replied, with a sincere but confused look. "Every day, every morning, as soon as I get up."

"Well I don't know," said Geshe Lothar, sounding a little dubious. He looked down in the general direction of the first flight of stairs and said, "I think some of these steps—down near the bottom, you see, might need a little touching up, you see, what with all the traffic coming and going," and he glanced at me.

"Yes Elder One, right away," replied the young monk pleasantly.

"Nawang, better get down there with your bucket before he does the steps, or you'll track dirt all over them again," said Geshe Lothar to the other boy. "Doesn't help to have fresh milk if there's no stream water to brew the tea right!" And the other monk groaned and got up to get the bucket.

"That ought to buy us some time," he smiled at me. "The stream is way out on the other side of the main gates. And besides that I just filled those two up with a big breakfast of mo-mo dumplings. Lunrik probably won't even be able to bend over to sweep, hee-hee!" he giggled, as the young monk went down the steps heavily, carrying one of those short little Tibetan hand-brooms.

Then Geshe Lothar's face turned serious and he made me sit down at the table. He took the lid off a small wooden bowl before him and sipped some tea slowly, while I frowned at the ground. "Looks pretty serious," he said finally. "Go ahead, you can tell me everything. Don't be afraid... Friday, isn't it?"

I nodded and gathered up my courage and then everything just poured out.

"Grandmother is very sick. She just lies there, like she's asleep, all the time. Nobody can help her. I remembered that night, the night you were going to tell me about the monster, the one with the big claws, in the painting of the Wheel of Life, and about the three bad creatures in the center, the ones who make people get sick and get old and die, people like Grandmother. And then the strange man in the white cloth came, the thread sage, and you didn't have a chance to tell me, and well, you see—now I really need to know, because Grandmother is really sick, and I really need to fix her. Just tell me how that Wheel works, and what I have to do, and I promise I'll do everything just right," I concluded with a confident nod.

Geshe Lothar raised an eyebrow and stared down at his bowl of tea. He began to frown a bit, and I started to get nervous. Then he looked across the table at me, dead serious, like a grown-up to a grown-up, and I was grateful.

"The first thing you need to know," he said, very deliberately, "is about that monster, the one with his claws around the Wheel. He is the Lord of Death."

I nodded seriously, but I didn't really understand. I hadn't really seen Death yet. Then I thought of something. "Where does he live?" I asked. "Does he ever look like... like a big terrible animal... almost like a really huge wild yak?"

Geshe Lothar accepted my question gracefully, and looked down and thought for a minute, and then raised his kind face again.

"Well, Friday, it's not exactly like that," and he paused again. Then he said, quietly, "The Lord of Death—you see—he's not really like that, like that picture. That's just to show how mean he is. Really he's just, well, part of everybody, inside everybody, from the day they are born.

"And in that first few minutes of your life, you see, he begins to eat away at your life—sort of like a rat, you see, inside—and he chews and chews from hour to hour, a little tiny bit at a time, and well then people start to get older, right then, from the very beginning, and then finally one day he's finished eating, and people just die."

I looked across to him for a while and absorbed all this, and he was kind enough to let me, in silence. Then I cleared my throat.

"And this monster, can you get him out of you? Can you get him out?"

Geshe Lothar—and I bless him deep in my heart every time I remember that moment—didn't even hesitate. "Of course," he said, telling me the truth of it with his eyes. "It is what we are here to do, it is all we really have to do."

"And the way to do it—the key—it has something to do with those three evil creatures, the ones in the very center of the Wheel?" I asked.

"Exactly," he nodded. "If you understand them, and the other little pictures in the Wheel—if you understand how all those parts work together, and how to work with them—then you can make the Lord of Death leave you forever."

I hesitated and thought for a moment. "And then do you just get older and older? I mean… do you just get like Grandmother and then even… older?"

"Oh no!" he laughed. "Who'd want to do that? No, you change—all of you changes—and your body then, it's like made of light, like the flame on top of a candle, all bright and gold."

I thought some more. "But can you still see all your friends, and your mother and your father, and your brother?"

"Of course!" he exclaimed.

"And are they like you too?" I asked.

"Of course!" he boomed back, almost indignantly.

"Then you must teach me about the Wheel of Life!" I gushed happily. Then I turned around and checked the sun. "I have about an hour before

I have to get going, back home..." I wavered. "I said I'd be back from the stream by lunch..."

Geshe Lothar smiled at my little confession. Then he looked down at his bowl once again and sighed softly. He reached out slowly, took it in his hand, and tilted it to the side, pouring a few drops of tea out onto the heavy plank of the table.

"Oh, I can tell you the words," he said softly. "It doesn't take long, although more than an hour; say a few days."

I nodded my agreement—I would find a way.

"But that's a little like pouring a few drops of tea on this big table here," he continued. He looked up at me sharply and squinted. "Put your hand under the table," he whispered, intensely. "Hold your palm up to the wood, tight."

I did it, and then he said "Feel the tea?"

I looked up at him with a growing sadness, because I felt where this was going.

"No," I answered simply.

He poured out another few drops. "Feel it now?"

159

"No," I replied, quiet, and I looked down sadly. We were silent for a moment.

"Friday, how long would it take me pouring little drops of tea before even just one drop soaked all the way through this big wood board and reached your hand?"

I pulled my palm away quickly and put it in my lap, and squeezed my hands together, and pushed them into my belly, feeling the impossibility of it.

"It's our heads, you see," he went on, gently. "Really hard!" and he rapped his knuckles on the side of his head, and made a funny look. It helped and I smiled.

"It takes time, Friday. A long time. You need to study for a long time, and you need a good teacher who will spend that long time with you, to help you. It goes in these little holes really fast," he jammed his fingers in his ears, "but then it has to cook there, sink in there, in your mind, for a long time, before it finally touches your heart, and then you know what to do.

"This is why the boys study to become a Geshe," he said, waving his arms at the rooms around us. "We want them to learn exactly what you want to learn, even though they maybe don't realize it's what they're learning, until later..." he paused again.

"It takes that long?" I was almost crying.

Geshe Lothar nodded. "In most cases," he said simply. "Of course there are special people," he added. "And special... ways." He gazed at me thoughtfully, and then spoke to me again in that grown-up way, and he spoke the truth.

"I'll put it to you bluntly, and you think on it, you think on it, and you don't forget your grandmother. People who want to stop Death have to learn a lot of what a Geshe learns. You need that understanding—people always need that first. And then they need to go be by themselves for a while, you see, and pray, and meditate, hard. And for that, I'll tell you a secret," he winked.

I gazed at him, spellbound.

"For that," he continued, "it helps a lot, it makes things go a lot faster, if you know some of the ways of the sages..." he paused. "...*The thread sages,*" he added, in a whisper, winking at me again.

"There are things the monks know that the sages used to know, and it seems like they forgot. But there are also things that the sages know that the monks used to know, but it seems like they forgot." And his whisper stopped there, and a soft wind came and carried his words away.

"Of course Vice-Abbots would never say things like this, and I'd really appreciate it if you kept that between us," he grinned.

I sat down for a good spell and digested again all that he had said.

"And then I can help Grandmother too?" I asked quietly, urgently.

"Ah that," he said, looking down again, the drops of tea. They were nearly gone, nearly sucked into the wood. "I won't lie to you, Friday. You can't take death away from somebody else, not just like that, or else I figure—wouldn't you figure— that people who already knew all this stuff, I mean, being nice people, like they'd have to be, they'd just go around quick and kick that old Lord of Death out of people right away, right?"

He looked across at me brightly, and I nodded in agreement. It made sense.

"So it seems like," he said, following the thought, "that it's something each one of us has to learn to do ourselves. Even your grandmother would have to learn, and she'd have to want to learn, and there'd have to be someone who really cared about her, to teach her."

He looked across at me again, his eyes bright, this time with almost-tears. "And that person, you see, that person would have to learn everything as fast and hard and sincerely as they could manage, and not just for their own grandmother, but for everyone around who might be willing and able to learn how to stop the monster.

"And that person would have to be really strong, and even if something happened to their grandmother—even if, say, she didn't wake up at all, and so she couldn't listen and learn what to do—even if she... died... before anyone could help her, well that person would have to just keep on going, and learn what they need to learn, because the world is full of other people too, who are all going to end up one day like Grandmother, you see, old and almost asleep, in that bed..."

15.

The World for a Jar of Water

There was a thump at the head of the stairs and the young monk stepped up, puffing, holding the broom in one hand and his tummy with the other. Geshe Lothar widened his eyes at me, a message.

"Well, I have to say, it tastes great!" he burst out, pointing to the jug. "Do you guess your Mommy would settle for two *ba-mos* of barley per jug?"

I thought fast. A *ba-mo* was a way we used to measure grain in the old days: you reached into a bag and scooped out as much as your hand could hold and well, that was a *ba-mo*, and it was like our money, and you bought things with *ba-mos* of grain.

"Depends on whose hand you use for the *ba-mo*," I shot back quickly. This was an expression I'd heard Grandmother use on Tuesdays, at the farmers' market in our nearby village of Kishong, for as long as I could remember. Geshe Lothar once told me later that the quickness of my reply was what made his mind up to help a seven-year-old girl embark on the course I was about to take.

"Fairly spoken," he laughed. "Oh Lunrik," he said to the boy off-handedly. "Did you catch the roof too?" Most Tibetan houses where we lived had a flat roof made of a special clay that we packed down really hard, over timbers, so you could walk up and stand on it and enjoy the evening or the stars. There were little walls around the edge to keep people, especially children, from falling off.

"The roof?" wheezed the boy.

"That's what I said,"

"But, Esteemed One, I swept it just yesterday... you were there," replied the young monk, respectfully.

"Ah yes," announced Geshe Lothar, "but those crows, you know! Such a mess!" and he made a face.

"Yes sir," and the boy trudged up a smaller staircase that led to the roof.

I had been thinking hard, and headed off whatever Geshe Lothar had intended to say next. "Well then it's all decided," I said firmly, another Grandmotherism. "The first step is that you must teach me the Geshe course, as soon as possible."

It was truly a sign of Geshe Lothar's greatness that he didn't even blink. He just looked me square in the eye for a moment and then said, "Friday, I know people are probably always telling you things like 'Girls don't do that'…"

A voice got ready to go off in my head.

"… so I'm not going to say that." The voice went back to sleep.

"But there's something you have to realize. There are certain monks who teach the classes around here, and then there are other monks who have to run the monastery so the other monks can teach the classes—you see?

"And me, I'm one of the second kind, I'm stuck trying to help run this place." He leaned towards me across the table and made a funny face and said, "And I can tell you, it's a r-r-r-real head-ache!" Then he let out a big laugh, and settled back on his seat, and gazed at me thoughtfully for a moment.

"But your uncle—isn't Geshe Jampa Rabgay your uncle? He's the greatest teacher this monastery has ever seen—that's why people tromp all the way out to your place for his classes! Why don't you get him to teach you?"

I made a little scowl and stared down at the top of the table. "He's a real nice man," I blurted out, "but he's such a green-brain!" This was a rather impolite way in our language to call someone old-fashioned; Geshe Lothar raised an amused eyebrow but I just raced on. "He won't let me study in his classes—he won't even let me walk into a class long enough to bring him a little churn of tea, and so Tenzing—that's my brother—he has to keep running back and forth between Uncle's yurt and the family yurt carrying the next cup of tea, and I bet Tenzing doesn't even hear half the class!" I found I was half up off the ground and then remembered myself and sat down with a plop, sulking a bit just at the memory of it.

"Hmm, I see," said Geshe Lothar. A mischievous look was growing on his face, as he stared at the little pool of tea left in his bowl, swirling it around. "Your family—you have a sweet lady who comes to milk the cows in the morning?" he mused.

"Yes, Bukla," I replied.

"My cousin, you know," he said, sort of lost in a thought. I smiled, because "cousin" is such a broad term in our language that almost everybody was cousins.

"Done, Venerable One! One hundred percent done!" and suddenly the pleasant little monk had appeared again, stepping down off the staircase that led to the roof.

"And well done!" boomed Geshe Lothar back, with a smile, his mind obviously made up on something. The young monk stepped over to the table and stood respectfully, ready I think to sweep the whole countryside around us if that were the next directive, but Geshe Lothar just laughed and waved his hand in my direction.

"Lunrik, I say, could you take that jug to the hearth, and pour the milk into a pot to heat and then give our visitor back her jug? She's got to be home pretty soon."

"Yes Venerable," and the boy leaned over and put out his hands to me. I caught Geshe Lothar with a quick sideways glance and made a very strong little shake with my head.

"Oh Lunrik," he burst out again, and the boy straightened. "Come to think of it, I think it's much more auspicious if the very first milk from this little lady's family were served to the entire Council of Elders at that next meeting—when was that, this coming Friday, isn't it?"

"Yes sir, just so, sir," replied the boy, and I breathed a little sigh of relief.

"Ah yes, Friday. Lucky day, Friday. That's perfect. So could I ask you, my little friend," and then Geshe Lothar began standing up from the table, "to return three days hence, on Friday, say a couple of hours before noon, and bring us another ah... *full...* jug of your best milk, for the meeting of the Council? They always get a special tea then, you know, served in those ridic... I mean, those *special* little porcelain cups! And I'll have all the other arrangements made by then, you see? And tell Mommy I agree to the two *ba-mos* and that we'll use the biggest hand around to measure them out!" And he looked all around dramatically and then thrust out his hand. "Mine!" he roared, and threw back his head with laughter. He took my hand and helped me up, with a curious little peer into the jug when Lunrik wasn't looking, and then turned to the young monk again.

"Little Venerable, I say, could you direct our friend to the main gates, and make sure she knows how to get back here, for Friday?"

"Yes sir," smiled the unbelievably obedient one, and he started ahead of me down the stairs.

I turned to Geshe Lothar but he just gave me a big wink that said absolutely everything was taken care of, and so I thanked him from my very heart with my eyes, and took a few steps down, my excitement growing. But then another of those questions jumped into my mind, and I turned around again. Geshe Lothar had his elbows up on the wall around the landing, looking over the monks' houses, off to the fields and the forest and the horizon, lost in thought.

"Er, Venerable One, Vice-Abbot, sir?" I called him back.

He seemed a bit startled but then turned and threw his big smile warmly all over me again. "Yes, Friday?"

"Just one last thing, you know. I... I was wondering. Why doesn't Uncle... I mean, why doesn't Uncle fix Grandmother?"

Geshe Lothar looked me right in the eyes again and said, matter-of-factly, "Maybe there's something *you* have to do."

We stood there like that in the shaft of sunlight with our eyes together, I remember. And then I nodded and hurried off after Lunrik.

16.

Plans are Laid

When Bukla showed up on Friday one of the cows seemed to have taken a little ill and wasn't giving much milk at all—and I had a warm, largish jug-full tucked away out behind the stone shrine, near the back path to the monastery. I went to play down at the big pool again until lunch and fairly skipped to the monastery, despite my load.

Geshe Lothar and his big sunny smile were there waiting for me and suddenly there were lots of chores inside for his two young helpers, and we were left at the big table on the landing again, in the glorious sun of a beautiful day.

"Now this is how it's going to go," began the Vice-Abbot, and then we had a long serious talk that I really promised never ever to tell anyone, even you, about.

Then we went into Geshe Lothar's amazing little room, sort of like a little piece of a Bengal jungle right there in the middle of Tibet, jammed full of neat things with even neater little things stashed all over. And he made Lunrik climb up on a stool and reach into all sorts of little nooks and crannies up near the ceiling and pull down dusty little pouches and boxes with wonderful things in them and he took a bit from here and a pinch from there and folded them in little pieces of cloth and tied them up with strings and stuffed them into my shoulderbag, spouting a steady flow of special instructions and making me repeat them back to him to make sure I had them right.

And then he unwrapped a very old exquisite piece of silk and pulled out a *tsa-tsa*. This is a little clay tablet with a picture of a holy being stamped onto it. And he told me it was Gentle Voice, the Angel of Wisdom, the same one that Di-di-la had mentioned when he explained how he got his name. And then Geshe Lothar taught me that special prayer for being able to understand your lessons better, and he made me repeat it over and over until he was certain it sounded just right.

And then he took my hand and made sure I had my jug of—milk—and led me off through the monks' houses towards the courtyard of the wisdom warriors. But before we reached the main wall we took a turn through several piles of logs and into a large darkish room with a high ceiling. I stared in wonder at the walls, covered with every kind of pot and pan and ladle and spoon imaginable, hanging from great iron hooks. Then I stared even longer at the monastery kettles—huge metal vats that could hold hundreds of cups of tea, set on low brick walls over massive pits filled with blazing fires.

"My old home," laughed Geshe Lothar, and suddenly I realized that both our faces were already nearly covered with sweat. "The monastery kitchen. Seven years running this place! Ah, the road to Vice-Abbot was long, and hard!" he sighed deeply.

"Master Cook!" he bellowed then. "Master Cook! Come out, come out, wherever you are!"

And then out from behind one of the big kettles in a dark corner appeared a quiet, humble old monk. He was very thin, as though most of his body had sweated away long ago over one of the great cooking fires. But his arms were all taut and woven into strong cords of muscle from stirring and lifting. He had soot smeared over most of his face, but it only made it sweeter when he greeted us with a huge smile.

"Yes Vice-Abbot sir! Oh magnificent one!" and he patted Geshe Lothar's big happy belly affectionately.

Geshe Lothar peered down at his tummy and said to me, "That's all *his* doing you know!"

The Master Cook gave me a friendly wink and said to Geshe Lothar, "What can I do for you two today? You can't possibly be hungry, not with the breakfast we served up this morning." Then he paused and said to me in a loud whisper, leering at Geshe Lothar's girth, "Well I suppose *some* people could still be hungry!"

Geshe Lothar hrrumphed. "Actually, Master Cook, this young lady has brought a jug full of very special milk to be used for the tea that's served at the meeting of the Council of Elders this afternoon. It's to be masala tea, with real sugar, you see."

The Master Cook gave him a surprised look. "Masala tea! Not much likelihood of that! I don't even lay eyes on spices like that more than, oh, once a year! Come all the way from the middle of India! How're we going to serve them masala tea?"

Geshe Lothar turned to me with a flourish and I began pulling little packets out of my shoulderbag, and the Master Cook's eyes got bigger and bigger as we opened them up; and then there was a long fun training session on the subtleties of brewing masala tea.

Then we excused ourselves, "Gotta run, Master Cook! We don't have to eat these here—we can just chew them on the way!" and Geshe Lothar reached behind a little curtain into a niche in the wall and pulled a couple of fresh *kapsay* pastries out of a pot there.

"Hey!" said the Master Cook.

"Really should think of a better place to hide them," snickered Geshe Lothar, as he popped one in his mouth, handed me the other, and bounced out the door.

I chewed happily and Geshe Lothar led me to a long building with all windows and no door that I could see. We went downhill, around the back, and there was a long covered porch, with one small wooden portal. He opened it and took my hand and we stepped into another world altogether.

I looked to my left; sun was pouring in through the windows on the opposite wall, and all I could see was row upon row of young monks, sitting on thick woolen carpets. Before each monk was a small wooden table; they were painted gaily with all different bright colors and had dragons and flying horses and stars and suns and moons carved all over the sides. On top there was a hole cut into the wood to accommodate a small clay pot of ink; each person had a bamboo pen in hand and was stooped over a long thin piece of rice paper, carefully covering it with strokes of elegant calligraphy.

Above this sheet, which was about as long as your hand and as wide as your whole arm, was another sheet, already covered with writing. There were several older monks walking quietly around the room, bending occasionally to whisper something or change a pot of ink. And there was one very old, very intense-looking monk wrapped in a rich woolen elder's cloak—he was working slowly up and down a wide aisle left between the rows, his neck and back ramrod-straight, like Grandmother's had been, and his crinkly old eyes staring around the room, like a hawk's. Everything was completely silent, but for the slight scraping noise of bamboo on paper.

"The scriptorium," whispered Geshe Lothar, "the place where we copy out the sacred books. One of the best in all Tibet. We make all our own paper too, and it's probably the finest anywhere." He nodded over to the right side of the room, and behind a curtain I could see another group of young monks—some setting huge squares of paper out to dry on a shelf in the sunlight; others almost up to their knees in long thin scraps of paper that fell as they cut pages out of the sheets of raw paper, using wooden clamps and razor-sharp knives.

"No joking here," warned Geshe Lothar, as the hawk-eyed elder caught sight of us and started down the aisle in our direction. "Old Grumpy there runs this place with an iron fist," whispered my guide.

Then Geshe Lothar straightened himself up all official-like and joined his palms before his chest, in a formal greeting to the old man. "Ah, Master Calligrapher. An honor to see you this fine morning."

The Master Calligrapher surveyed this formality with a frank bit of suspicion, glancing down at me as well. "And Vice-Abbot, sir! To what do we owe the honor! Not often we see you in these parts!"

Geshe Lothar pulled the Master Calligrapher slightly off to the side and they held a whispered conference. Young monks were glancing up curiously and I just stared at the ground and tried to listen in. I heard Geshe Lothar say stuff like "Grandmother... royal family... Northerner," and then "possibility, you know, of a major donation" and then "new wing on the main temple" and finally "just a few little scraps, play along, you know, probably just wants to stuff a doll or something." It occurred to me that listening to Geshe Lothar talk about Grandmother was a lot like listening to Grandmother talk about Geshe Lothar.

And then the two men turned around to me and the Master Calligrapher gave me a kind of funny long thin smile and said, "Well, I'm sure our little visitor would appreciate a brief tour of what is probably the most important place in the whole monastery." And then it seemed like forever that he was leading us along through row after row of monks crafting their masterpieces, lecturing Geshe Lothar and me on all the fine points of the art of the scribe: describing the minerals used for the inks; the proper cut of the bamboo pens; and — most glorious of all — the names and contents of the various books that were being copied that very morning.

I was in a complete trance. I had seen the special books that Uncle was singing for our family every night, but I had honestly never thought much about how they were made or who made them. In fact I had never seen people write much at all, really only Uncle, and then usually only when Father needed a formal letter written to someone for his business.

You see, I know it sounds strange to you, but in our monasteries knowledge has always been passed on mainly by what we call "lips to ear" — meaning that the teacher would explain things to the students and they would listen really hard in this special way that we learned so that, you see, we would remember just about everything the teacher said as soon as they said it. And they were usually explaining a book from ancient times that almost everyone in the monastery had already memorized, every single word, one after the other, exactly, without a single mistake. And so books weren't so much something that was written down in letters, but more of a thing that was contained in like a song, and that song was passed down very carefully, without any changes at all, from generation to generation. And in a way it was more safe than books — you could never lose the book, because the book was there all the time, in your head, and you could take out a little piece whenever you wanted to, wherever you happened to be, and sing it out loud or just sing it in your mind, to yourself, and think about what it meant.

And so of course we had fewer books than people do nowadays, because it takes a while to memorize a whole book, and there are only so many books your mind can hold; but all the books we did have were really important ones, full of wonderful and very precious things like the teaching on the Wheel of Life — how to stop sickness, and getting old, and death itself, you see. And so what I mean to say is that we didn't write that much, but in many ways that was a better thing, and many of the old wise ones considered written books almost like using a crutch when your legs were fine anyway: they just sort of get in the way and make your real legs—your mind—weaker if you depend on them too much, instead of putting the book in your own memory. And if you really learn the old sacred ways, then your memory, and your mind, can hold tons more than you would guess.

But lots of people, and I guess you could say Uncle was one of the main ones where we lived, realized all the other very real benefits that could come from writing certain things down, as long as it didn't get distracting. And so all the young monks were taught to read, and they had built the scriptorium, and as I walked around I felt the power of what was happening there. I also knew that, to tell you the truth, very very few women were ever taught to write. But I turned to the Master Calligrapher anyway, and exclaimed, "Oh sir, could I just try it once, just once? Could you just show me to do anything, like just one letter?"

Geshe Lothar looked a little worried, but the Master Calligrapher's love of his art had already overwhelmed his annoyance at our interruption. He shuffled us up to his desk in the front, and called over one of the assistants. They exchanged a few words and the assistant left—and then I was sitting at the huge big beautiful desk in the sunlight, on the cushion of the Master Calligrapher himself, and he was leaning over me and I could smell a fragrance coming from him like ink and sandalwood and jasmine all mixed together, and his old steady hand was wrapped around my tiny fingers, and a fine, worn bamboo pen was there, and we dipped it into a little pot and he guided my hand over the lovely touch of the paper and then there was:

And I whispered in sheer excitement "Oh what is it, what is it?" And he felt the energy coming up through my hand and he whispered back, with the same excited awe, "It is *ja*, little one. It is the word for 'tea'."

And I sat up straight and looked at my first letter, overcome with pride and almost a kind of reverence, and then—I don't know why—I started to cry, for happiness. And the two monks looked down at me, and then at one another, silently, for the longest time.

And then the assistant was back, and he had a good-sized cloth bag in his hands, and it was filled with the long thin scraps of paper that had covered the floor where the cutters were working. And he handed it to the Master Calligrapher, who turned and stooped and put it in my arms gently and said, "This is for you, my friend. For stuffing your dolls, or..." and he gave Geshe Lothar an odd ironic look, "... or whatever." And then he rummaged around in the drawer and pulled out a little sachet and set it in the bag too, quietly.

I turned and looked up at his face, and his eagle eyes were glistening. "Ink powder," he said gruffly. "Add water. Clean water. Not too much."

And then it was over and he straightened up with the look of someone who has to get back to work, and Geshe Lothar said "Thank you" for both of us, and I walked almost all the way home with the Master Calligrapher's favorite pen before I realized it was still in my hand, but then I felt his hand around mine again, guiding it through the one letter, and I knew he had given it to me then.

17.

I Become a Milkmaid

I sprang our trap on the family a few days later, on Sunday, and I must say it went absolutely perfectly. After Bukla had milked the cows she came in and asked Amala if she could have a word, and Amala gave me a look that told me to go outside and play. Grandmother was still the same and it seemed like people were hardly noticing her, except for some soup and cleaning her messes a few times a day. Father was out on caravan. I stepped outside and positioned myself where I figured the action would be taking place.

I heard sort of a strained exchange between Amala and Bukla through the flap over the yurt door, and then the milkmaid came out with a bit of a long face, but threw a warm glance in my direction. I knew it would take a few minutes more and I fidgeted around until Bukla was out of sight and then—on schedule—Amala stepped quietly from the yurt out into the clearing, calling "Jampa! Oh Uncle Jampa!"

Uncle came out quickly, Tenzing trailing after him. "Is something wrong? Is it Grandmother?" he asked in a worried voice.

"Not Grandmother; it's Bukla!" exclaimed Amala, throwing her hands up in the air. "She's leaving! I can't believe it! Says she has to go right away! I can't believe it!"

"Go?" said Uncle, distractedly. "Go where? What's happened?"

"Says she can't milk the cows anymore! Says that she'll be too busy! Says the monastery has sent word, asking if she'd like to supervise the monastery dairy, down the hill from the monastery! Says she'll be in charge of six milkmaids herself! I can't believe it!"

Uncle held up his palms trying to find something comforting to say, but in truth I'm not sure it had ever occurred to him—between his books and his classes—that anyone ever milked the cows.

"Says she'll be back this evening, with her husband!" rattled on Amala. "To pick up her milk jugs! Says we can keep some until we get our own! I can't believe it!" she cried.

Uncle opened his mouth but Amala wasn't finished. "I can't do everything myself," she wailed. "I can't spin the yarn, with Grandmother the way she is now, and weave the carpets too, and do all the cooking, and look after the cows and do the milking and…" she started to cry "… and make everyone tea all day long."

At this last part, Uncle's eyebrows finally shot up in concern. Books? Classes? Prayers and meditation? Without tea? I could see his mind working furiously. I let the tension build for a few more seconds and then I stepped right between those two poor grown-ups and showed them how it was going to be.

"*I,*" I said, "I will be milking the cows." They stared down at me and I nodded with authority, like Grandmother. Uncle looked over at Amala, but she was a little stunned. "*And,*" I continued, "I will be letting them out to pasture." Then there was more stunned silence.

"Grandmother taught me a long time ago how to spin the yarn, and I will be doing that in the afternoons," I announced further. "Here is a bagful I've been working on," and I pulled it out and handed it to Amala. She had recovered and—

rather than objecting, as I'm sure Grandmother would have done—she actually gave me a frankly grateful look.

"Now since I'll be milking the cows, I will also be making the tea," I went on firmly. "I will do so on a little fire over next to the cattle pens, so I can also see down to the pastures and stream, and check on the cows regularly. Probably best to make a ring of stones over there," I pointed towards the back of Uncle's yurt, "so Tenzing doesn't have so far to go when he comes to get Uncle's tea. That way he won't miss out on any of his classes." I smiled up at Tenzing, and he looked a little dubious, as in fact did everyone, for tea is something very sacred to Tibetan people, and it has to be done right. But I had expected this reaction, and waited patiently for the grown-ups to walk into the second phase of the trap.

"Well, I don't know about that last part," said Uncle, a little uncertainly, looking up at Amala and checking in with her.

"Yah," blurted Tenzing. "That could be a problem…"

"But you're just a child,…" sighed Amala sadly. "Why, you can't even reach the top of the big churn."

When everyone was finished I put my hands on my hips and faced them with my best Grandmother look. "Well, there's one way to find out, isn't there?" I declared.

"Today, I will make the afternoon tea. And if it's not the best tea you three have ever tasted here at the homestead, well, then I'll stick to yarn and cows. Agreed?"

They just looked at me with their jaws a little ajar and I nodded firmly. "It's all decided then. And Tenzing," I said, as I turned back to the family yurt. "I'll need at least a small fire over there behind Uncle's, say about an hour after lunch." I didn't wait to see his reaction. Best to get them used to having me over near Uncle's from the very start, I thought, as I walked to the door. And from the silence behind me I knew I at least had my chance.

The sun was still hanging a good three hours above the stone ridge when I was almost done with the tea. Tenzing kept finding excuses to be walking to and fro, from Uncle's to the family yurt. Amala peeked out a couple of times and I was careful not to notice. Even Uncle made a lot more trips to the toilet than he ever had before.

I just pretended I was the Master Cook—it was easier since I'd already gotten soot all over myself. I scalded the milk the right amount, and threw in pinches of the different spices, each at their own appointed time. At the very end, the plunger was a bit of a challenge, but I'd already set up one of Amala's weaving stools. I got up on top of it and pushed and pulled with sheer determination. Grandmother wasn't that far away, I thought to myself, just on the other side of the felt wall of the family yurt.

I poured my final product out into a serving kettle and tasted a bit, like I'd seen the Master Cook do. Then just to show off (feeling various eyes on my back), I opened one of the packets at random and tossed in an extra pinch of spice. And then I walked around the clearing with a regal stride like Grandmother would have done, collecting my three hapless charges and herding them towards my new spot behind Uncle's yurt. They looked a little nervous as I poured out a small steaming cup for each. They sipped. And then they sipped again. Silence. And then Tenzing gulped down all the rest of his and let out a big Ahhh!

"No question at all about it," he said, smacking his lips and giving me his I-can't-believe-you-did-it look. "Best cup of tea I've ever tasted here."

Uncle had gulped his tea down too, and began to blurt out something, but then thought better of it—paused—and glanced sheepishly over towards Amala. Tibetan women take great pride in their tea.

"Well it certainly is quite delicious," he admitted. "And I think you could say," he added in a diplomatic tone, "that it's the best cup of *this particular type of tea* I've ever had here.

"Much different from our normal salt-and-butter tea, you see," he continued, covering himself further, like someone in a debate at the courtyard of the wisdom warriors. "In fact, quite a lot like a tea I had just recently, down at the monastery, in a meeting of the Council of Elders," he mused, and shot me a quizzical look.

I let the look fly right past me and turned to my mother. "What do you think, Amala?" This deal had to be closed, soon, before anyone could think of why it shouldn't be.

"I think," she said, pouring a rare smile over me, and hugging my shoulder warmly, "I think we have not only a new milkmaid, but a new teamaker in this family."

I hugged her back with a very loud "Oh, wonderful!" And then, as if—on cue—a loud cheerful voice said, "Well, I couldn't have chosen a better replacement myself!"

And there was Bukla, coming around the side of Uncle's yurt. At her side was her husband, Norbu, a tall handsome man from the Eastern Provinces. He was a skilled carpenter and leather-worker who often accompanied Father on caravan. His eyes were bright and happy, and he had long black hair tied up around his head. From his ears hung small turquoise earrings—all in a style that was popular with those fiercely independent nomads in our days. Behind him followed a fine black horse with a bright braided bridle of yak hair, and large leather saddlebags.

"Come have some tea," I cried to them, "there's plenty for everyone." And we all huddled around the fire in the afternoon and shared our happiness. Bukla chattered on the whole time, about her new job down the hill from the monastery, and then filled us in on the latest news about what the monks were up to. She led the family very gradually around to phase three of the plan.

"And you see, there's been some decision by the senior Lamas—it seems like they've asked all the monks, especially the teachers, to add more windows to their rooms, so that the spirits of the land who are always roaming about will hear all the sweet words of the classes and the prayers, and then they won't mind so much when the monastery starts to spread out a bit next year, because they're planning some new dormitories and such," she said.

Uncle, poor man—Could he see what was coming? Did he have any choice?—cupped his hands around his tea and looked dreamily into the fire. "Why yes," he nodded. "That very same thing came up at the meeting of the Council of Elders, a few days ago…"

"… Oh yes," rushed on Bukla, seizing the moment. "And so Norbu here, he's been busy as a bee going from house to house down at the monastery, knocking out holes in the walls and setting up window frames and thick flaps to cover them for the cold weather. Haven't you, Norbu?" I saw her elbow poke the taciturn young man.

"Yup, yup," he agreed. Another elbow—ah, just right, my wonderful Bukla. "Your new window would go well right up here," he nodded towards the back of Uncle's yurt, and smiled at the unsuspecting scholar.

"New… window? A window in a yurt?" spluttered Uncle.

"Oh of course," Bukla flowed on. "Why Norbu just finished one, on the way here, for that old hermit who lives in a yurt over near the little tea shop, on the horse road, didn't you ..."

No extra elbow needed; Norbu was getting the hang of it. "Yup, yup," he agreed. "Came out right nice, with a nice cover against wind and rain. Can't believe nobody thought of it before..."

Bukla shot him one last look.

"And you know, it goes right quick!" he added. "Hardly takes an hour! Happen to have all the tools and stuff right here in our saddlebags!"

And then Amala, bless her heart, she was in such a relieved mood that she took it all over right there, and Uncle was walking around scratching his head, and the window was finished (well after sunset, to tell the truth), and since Tenzing didn't have anything else to do with all that sawing and pounding going on, why then Amala even put "my little Geshe" to work, lugging big rocks here and there.

And so the next morning found me in my new domain, with jugs and a nice big table and a wonderful new fireplace and the big tea churn and assorted kettles and—most important of all—a magic window to the world of Uncle's classes, right behind my head as I churned the tea.

18.

Those Who Listen

So now the cows got milked at the same exact time that Tenzing's class got their lessons, and I heard every word, through the window. My studies took on a life of their own—I had begun them in order to find a way to help Grandmother, but I soon grasped that it was that and something bigger too: a way I could help everyone in my small world. I saw a pattern in the lessons, and in the books. It was all like one of Amala's big carpets—pictures scattered all over from corner to corner, but each of them woven into one huge whole that could be picked up and offered to anyone who would accept the gift. And I also saw, sadly, that it would take time—maybe a long time—for this particular weaving to be finished. Maybe more time than Grandmother had.

Grandmother Tara had slowly worsened; it became very hard to get any food into her, even soup, and she grew more and more thin. But that wasn't the worst thing, not at all, and I knew what was. It was how she changed for us, for all of those who truly loved her. Slowly, imperceptibly, we left her, each of us, the way that she was leaving us—I suppose, to be honest, it was *because* she was leaving us.

People paid her less and less attention, and then finally came the day when it was decided—I don't think by any one of us, but just by all of us—to move her over to a yurt of her own. The caravan men brought it in on a pair of horses—a yurt is really just a pile of poles and a covering, which is what makes them so useful, so easy to carry, so easy to put up, so easily broken down and swept away, at the end. They had it up in less time than it had taken to cut Uncle's window, out on the edge of the clearing where the path to the horse road started. And so now we had three yurts, in sort of a triangle.

Amala and I took turns going over to check on Grandmother—feeding her what we could, cleaning her up, stoking the fire. No one ever admitted it, but we were all relieved when the smell that had sunk into her clothes and mattress was gone from the family yurt. Amala directed moving over all of Grandmother's things, and we were very respectful and careful with the little possessions—

the *nice things*—that she had loved so much. But she was oblivious to them all, and woke or slept the same in their midst, staring out the new sky window at the same blue sky. And we all felt terribly guilty to have moved her, as I suppose families do and should everywhere, and the big empty space on the side of the family yurt reminded us of this particular cruelty of life over and over, especially at night—when the dark and the half-conscious times around sleep raised doubts.

Finally Amala set up a big loom, with a half-finished carpet of different lovely scenes, in the space where Grandmother had been. It helped a bit, but the place still seemed broken and incomplete—the same as our sense of family. I felt strangely vulnerable when I slept, without Grandmother on the one side to match Father and Amala on the other, protecting us. But I had Tenzing, and he was growing still stronger and more handsome and intelligent and cheerful by the day. No one had a better brother, or teacher.

For one day I finished the tea early and had a few extra minutes before the break between classes—that was when I was supposed to set the small churn, hot and full, on the little shelf that Bukla's husband had built below Uncle's window. I was sitting by myself next to the fire, practicing the one letter that the Calligraphy Master had taught me, writing it in the dirt with a stick. And so on a whim, when I put the churn on the shelf, I wrote the letter — which is also the word for "tea" — there in the dust on the shelf, turned upside down so the other person could read it better:

And then I went on with my business as usual, for my days had become much more full. I returned after two more classes had left — not even thinking about the letter — to collect the churn and refill it. I came and grabbed it and almost didn't notice that something new was written in the dust on the shelf. This time it was turned around to face me:

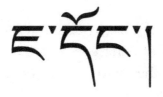

I stood riveted on the letters for a long time, the churn still up there on the shelf, clasped in my hands. I thought furiously. I had a feeling that the big slash on the end was just a way to announce that a sound or word was finished, so that wasn't so hard. Another full three or four minutes passed before I finally looked up at the churn in my hands and realized that this had to be the word for tea-churn: *ja-dong*. But I wasn't all that sure about the little dots—maybe they did something, or maybe they were just random smudges. I determined to squeeze it out of Tenzing after we settled down for sleep that night.

"Tenzing, dear brother?" I asked, when Amala's breathing had slowed into sleep, and we had put our heads close together, there on the floor before the family fire, for our nightly talk.

"Yes Friday, my precocious little sister," he replied, and I'm sure he knew what was coming.

"If someone was trying to write a word, let's say 'tea-churn,' and there was a lot of extra dots and stuff all over the place, well—how would they know which was which?"

"Girls don't do that—girls don't learn to write," he answered back bluntly; not to be mean, you know, but I think to make sure my stubbornness would rise and make me take his lessons seriously.

I kicked him hard in the shin, under the covers, and he yelped—just once—and by the time Amala's breathing had gone back to softness he was holding my palm, in the dark, covering it with the magic of new letters and their mysteries: why one letter could be quiet in a word but still needed to be there, why some had to have those little dots as friends, stuff like that. Another dam across the stream of my life was smashed down, at that moment, and the rushing waters of ideas—holy ideas, ideas that could help people like Grandmother—had a new place to flow now: across the paper, and from there into my heart.

It wasn't long before the words started piling up and the spaces on the shelf ran out. Drom and Stick and Hammer were also getting suspicious of the time that Tenzing and I spent at the window, and we didn't need any more trouble from them. Grandmother's sickness had just about stopped my visits to the courtyard of the wisdom warriors—Amala could never be persuaded to go unless Father was in town and in the mood—but I gathered from the talk between Tenzing and his friend Di-di-la that the debates between them and the little gang were becoming more and more intense. I couldn't afford to give them any more reasons to tease my brother, in front of everyone.

And so one day I went and got one of the
scraps of paper the Calligraphy Master had so
kindly given me. Grandmother Tara had always
said that the best place to hide something was right
out in front of everyone, so I'd stuffed the bag full
of scraps into the cushions I used for a pillow, and
left it out there in the middle of the floor of the
family yurt. Amala was turned toward the wall
weaving, and I made small talk and pulled out a
piece, along with the pen and ink powder. I took it
all over to my little fire and sat close to the wall of
Uncle's yurt so no one could see, mixed up some
ink in a little clay dish, and laboriously wrote out:

ཉན་ཅན།

Which means, "I'm listening!" And I
slipped it under the tea churn on the next pass.

When I came back in the afternoon for the
churn I was shaking with excitement to see if
Tenzing had written me back. And I found the

same piece of paper waiting for me, with what I'd written changed around, like this

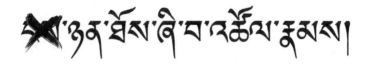

I swiftly whisked the paper into my palm and went on filling up the churn, my heart pounding. Then I walked over to Grandmother's, went in quietly, and sat down next to her in front of the little altar that every Tibetan home has somewhere. I gazed over at her with love—this time her eyes were closed, and she was sleeping softly—and in the same moment I wished I already knew enough to do something real to change her sickness; but I also felt how proud she'd be if she knew how much I had already learned, out of the sheer stubbornness I'd studied from her.

I bent over the paper and slowly worked out the sounds there. And then something inside me broke—knowing I was getting close but maybe still too far away to ever help the dear woman at my side—and I cried over the paper, and the Master Calligrapher's fine ebony ink smeared all over everything—but even years later I could still read what was written there, and it was the first words of the first holy book I had ever learned:

Those who listen, seeking peace...

19.

The Hand with the Claws

From that day on, there was a little scrap of paper waiting for Tenzing under the tea churn every day they had classes. On it I had copied out, from memory, the lines he had written for me the day before. These he passed to me in the afternoon, on the back of the morning's paper—with all the letters I'd written checked and fixed for me. The lines were always the ones that the boys had all memorized for that particular day's lesson: usually a verse, or two, from what Tenzing (and I) were singing in the evening.

"Tenzing, dear brother," I asked one night, "how did you ever think to write me that first line, the one about those who listen?"

"You not only talk too much during the day," he groaned, rolling over, "but you also talk in your sleep."

I punched him in the back, but his answer was already on the way. "Don't worry, my little-girl Geshe," he chuckled. "It's very soft. And no one in here but me would understand what you were saying anyway. Now go to sleep!"

I don't know how my wonderful brother ever managed all the notes without Uncle and the class bullies catching on—but he did it. For my part, I began to spend more and more time with Grandmother, in the evening, and there in the light of the little butter-lamp on her altar I'd practice my writing. There too I'd sing the prayer that Geshe Lothar had taught me, to the Angel of Wisdom, to make my mind and my heart stronger. I think Grandmother could hear it—she was beginning to breathe very strangely most of the time, a kind of hoarse rasping sound, but whenever I sang the soft sounds of Gentle Voice her breath would begin to go slow and soft, nearly in time with the song.

Tenzing, on his evening rounds to sing the books he was committing to memory, had taken to going in a big circle around all three yurts. They had cut a window in Grandmother's yurt too—on the side, facing the path to the horse road—and so as my brother passed with his song I would sing along softly. I thought of it as a gift to her, to the one who had shown me the courage to try what I was trying, and as her breathing became gentler I felt she was accepting the gift.

One day—Father was home—Amala came back from feeding Grandmother Tara all quiet, and sobbing. And Father went out and Uncle came in with Tenzing and he said we would sit together by the fire for a while and I didn't know why but something felt terribly wrong and Amala tried to stop but she couldn't and she sobbed and sobbed, with a little whine sometimes that sounded like a small animal when it was really hurt.

And I don't know how long we spent like that but Uncle absolutely refused to let me and Tenzing leave the yurt, and then Father came back to get something out of one of his boxes and when he went to leave and opened the door again I looked and saw two men out there. One was big and strong and had sort of a blank look like a big ox, and he was carrying ropes and a big piece of cloth.

But it was the other man that frightened me; he was short, and very thin, and had greasy black hair that came down over his face, and his face too was dark and thin. And Father counted out something and thrust it towards the thin man. And the thin man put out his thin bony hand and clutched at what Father had handed, and I gasped.

"What is it, Friday?" said Uncle, turning around. I pointed to the door but just then the flap came down.

"That man," I said, my voice shaking. "The skinny one. I think he is the Lord of Death. He has those same claws, those same long claws that the Lord of Death has. I saw them in the picture of him, the one in the Wheel of Life."

Uncle opened his mouth to say something but then changed his mind and just turned and looked glumly into the family fire. Amala's sobbing got quieter and quieter, like it was going into her and now she was crying all on the inside.

And then finally Father came in and sat down next to Amala and put his arm around her. He turned to Tenzing and me and I saw this sincere look come all over his face, the same look I'd seen on Father's face once when he was trying to sell an old horse to a man from the village. And then Father began a long story about how Grandmother must have decided to go away, to be with some of her friends, probably sky people from her own place, and she would be really happy there with them, and Tenzing and I didn't need to worry about her a bit or be sad at all. And at the end

Tenzing said "Yes, Father," like the good heart that he was. But I couldn't say anything and I just glanced up at Father in a kind of rage because I didn't believe at all that Grandmother had gone anywhere that she wanted to go. I didn't believe that that elegant beautiful intelligent woman would lie in a bed for weeks covered in her own messes if she could have just gotten up and gone somewhere else any time she'd wanted to. And I especially didn't believe she would ever go away like that without talking to me a lot about it first and probably leaving me a whole pouch of dried cheese, for until she got back.

And what I did believe was that something very bad had happened, something that nobody had wanted to happen, something that nobody— not even any grown-up, not Father and not even Uncle—could control or stop. And I believed that it had something to do with the Lord of Death, because even if that skinny man with the evil look was not the Lord of Death himself, he had to be very close to him. And so I never said a word that day to Father; I just got up, and no one stopped me, and I went out to sit by myself at the stone shrine.

And then later on they held a big prayer for Grandmother in the main temple at the monastery, and all the monks came and sang for her together, and Father I suppose must have spent a lot of money, because every monk had a big nice meal there, and got some things like shoes or cloth for robes. And the prayer started in the afternoon, and they dressed me and Tenzing up all nice for it, but then when it was time to go I ran to Grandmother's, and I sat there on the floor in front of the altar and the empty bed, and Father and Uncle both came and tried to get me to come, but I wouldn't, I couldn't—I didn't believe I could help Grandmother that way. Maybe the others could, but I knew what I had to do. And they talked to me for a long time and I wouldn't even look at them, and Father bent over and looked like he might carry me all the way to the monastery, but Uncle put his hand on his arm and they looked—brother to brother—in each other's eyes for a long time, and finally Father just nodded.

And they all went away, and I ran and got my bag of paper scraps and came to be near Grandmother's things at least and lit a few small butter lamps to help her find her way, and then for her I sat down with that blessed pen and I began to write out all the blessed words I knew, all the lines Tenzing had ever taught me to write, I wrote one by one on the thin little scraps of paper. And all the time I cried, and every time I finished a line the paper was all wet and soggy with tears, and I would set that line carefully on the altar to help Grandmother—to tell her I was sorry that I hadn't learned enough, quickly enough, to help her really.

And I went on crying and writing as long as I could for her, into the night, and when at last what was left of our family came home Father came in and found me asleep in the papers and tears and carried me to bed, and never said a thing about it later. And when I woke up the next morning it was already late and the sun and the bright blue sky were pouring in through the sky-window and there was a funny bump in the floor under my shoulder and I turned over and there was Grandmother's little red pouch, all filled to the brim with pieces of dried cheese.

20.

It Will Not Be All Right

Three years passed then, quickly, because I was working hard. It wasn't just for Grandmother any more—I hadn't forgotten Geshe Lothar's advice, and I knew I had to go on, not only go on, but fly on, as fast and as strong as I could, to help everyone like my Grandmother—which might be everyone I knew.

I could stretch out the milking enough every day to catch most of Tenzing's class, and then he would fill me in on a lot of the rest during our late-night talks laying at the family fire. I caught on to a lot of the special language that the wisdom warriors used—just through the window, as Uncle grilled the young men. But I could rarely get to the courtyard, since a girl my age was expected to walk on the roads at night only with an adult, and Drom and his toughs were bound to tell on me to Uncle if they saw me there at the wall, alone.

Nobody had the heart to touch Grandmother Tara's things, and there was after all that story about her having gone to visit the sky people, and so by common consent her yurt became a beautiful little chapel that the whole family could use. Father gave me lots of pieces of lovely cloth to brighten up the altar, and I took care to keep it clean. I set the little clay picture that Geshe Lothar had given me—the one of Gentle Voice, the Angel of Wisdom—up on top wrapped in some little pieces of gold silk like angel robes. Then every day I put out little bowls of fresh clean water from the stream, because we believe that some of the nicest gifts you can give are just little things that come free from nature: things like stream water, or wild flowers, or even just your memory of the sunset from the evening before.

I also kept Grandmother's little red pouch up on the altar; just in case it did happen that she came back one day when I wasn't in the chapel, I knew she'd know I was still expecting her. I made new cheese every week or so and dried it into little squares and changed the ones in the pouch, so they'd always be the freshest, for her.

Drom and his gang were just as miserable as ever—they knew I was often in the chapel, and they passed by the little window every day coming down the path from the horse road. I guess they knew I could hear them, and it seems they had some pretty good guesses about my trying to do what a girl had never ever done; and so there were always some snide remarks floating through Grandmother's window when class let out.

"Wonder if Di-di-la's been able to get her to remember a whole line of that wisdom prayer yet?"

"Yah, what is it? Oh I forget!"

"I'll give you a clue! (Here they let me imagine one of them imitating Di-di-la's buck teeth and big scared eyes.)

"Oh yah! Di-di-di-di-di-di-di!" And then a roar of laughter.

One night when I was ten years old—to tell you the truth I don't remember a lot of any one day from those years, but this day is still as clear as today—Tenzing and I had finished going over the lessons there on our rugs in front of the fire. And Father and Amala were fast asleep, and the little butter lamps on the altar were sending their little rays of bright golden light across the family yurt, and I was falling into sleep myself, in that unmistakable warmth and contentment of a full day of doing things that were good, and would be of help to other people. And then Tenzing turned to me.

"Friday, are you still awake?" he whispered, and he seemed a little nervous.

"Yes," I said sleepily.

"Friday, I want to show you something. There's something you have to see."

"Okay, Tenzing," and I opened my eyes.

And then he reached down and pulled the covers aside. And he pulled up his undershirt, the one that all the monks wear under the top part of their robes, and use as pajamas at night too. And there was his beautiful, strong slender body in the light of the lamps and the fire. I blushed a little because I'd never really seen him like that, just glimpses sometimes when he was in the yurt and changing his shirt, and he would always turn away. But here was his lovely form.

"Here, look here," he said softly, and he pointed to his strong flat stomach. I propped myself up on one elbow and looked down—the light wasn't very good, it was all shadows. And then I saw a tiny little lump, only about the size of a small nut. It wasn't much at all. But somehow it looked very wrong. It didn't belong there, on my brother.

"Here, I want you to touch it," he said, and inside I blushed even stronger, because I had never touched Tenzing like that before.

But he took my little hand in his and pulled it down and made me touch it, with my finger. And then I drew my hand away, and he said, "I just wanted you to know, I wanted you to see it and touch it yourself, so you wouldn't be afraid."

"It is something bad," I said. It was not a question.

Tenzing paused and then said to me, in a firm voice, "Bad, but not so bad I think. Uncle's all worried about it, trying to make a big deal about it. But I'm not worried. I'm not going to let it hurt me. It will be all right, you'll see."

And I nodded and looked up at his face in the glow from the embers of the family fire, and I knew there was something he wasn't saying, and I got a little scared then, and I laid down and closed my eyes but I couldn't fall asleep, because I kept wondering why Tenzing had wanted so much for me to see and touch the thing and not be afraid of it if there was nothing to worry about, and it would be all right.

Then weeks and months flew by and we were all busy and happy with our lives. The classes leaking out the window of Uncle's yurt were wonderful; each new idea was like a brick for building a new house, and I would carry it over and add it to the ones I already had and soon I began to see a larger picture—how they all fit together into sturdy handsome walls, rising higher by the day. And so what I had begun almost in desperation I continued in nearly a leisurely satisfaction, for a while.

Tenzing never showed me the lump again and it laid there, hidden under his shirt, and a part of me would wonder and worry sometimes—if it was still there, if it was getting bigger, if it hurt. But he never said anything.

And then after about six months we were lying on the rugs at night talking quietly and it was hot and we had most of the covers thrown off and he was lying on his back, and the moonlight came in the sky-window and for some reason I looked down and my breath caught in my chest with fear, because I could see that the little bump had grown, and grown a lot, and now it was pressing up against Tenzing's undershirt.

And then one day a few weeks later the cruel boys, those cruelest boys, walked by

214

Grandmother's window, and one of them said, "Did you hear? Mommy's Little Geshe has a new nickname!"

"Oh too bad!"

"Yah! I really liked the old one!"

"Well tough luck, because it's no good any more! He's not little any more! Now he's *Druluk:* Mr. Potbelly!"

And they walked off laughing and didn't realize—I think they couldn't have realized, could they?—how much they had hurt me. And when I came out to the clearing that evening I watched Tenzing walk across to the family yurt and yes I could see that now his stomach was starting to swell out, and you could tell it, even under all of his robes.

And he never complained and he went on teaching me with extra devotion every single night. And whenever the wisdom warriors gathered he pulled himself up and down the road, even when the swelling got as big as a small melon, and his skin and his face were all turning gray and he couldn't speak a whole sentence any more without choking on something that came up.

And Amala, at first she was very worried, and I could hear her over near Uncle's yurt sometimes, asking questions almost hysterically, and Uncle's quiet, sad replies. And then one day she just got all quiet and went on with her weaving with a silent fervor and fussed over her little Geshe just like before, as if it would be all right, as if it were already all right.

And then one night sleeping there I dreamed I was in some other country altogether. And we were at the side of a huge, silent, strong river, a river so big I could hardly see across to the other side. And there was a whole group of us, and we were dressed all in beautiful soft long white cotton gowns, that wrapped around us as if we were angels.

And I was crying, crying and crying out in my grief, and there was a stone platform there up on a little hill, and it was painted white. And on top of the platform was a huge bed of wooden sticks and logs. And it was burning, and the golden flames were flying high into the air as the sun went down.

And there was a powerful smell, a smell of flesh burning, a great cloud of the smell and the smoke spreading into the evening air. And I was fighting to get away from the women around me but they were holding me back by the arms and I strained ahead with all my might and then there, laid out on the bed of the fire, there was my dear brother Tenzing, and he was dead and wrapped in his robes—different robes—robes of a sort of saffron mixed with pink, and the robes were burning and he was burning.

And I bolted up full awake and it was terribly dark in the yurt and there was that same terrible smell of burning flesh and smoke filling the whole room and I cried, "Father!" and he woke up and went to the altar and lit one of the small lamps and there, in that feeble light, was my beautiful brother, lying across the stone floor on his side, with his head all cocked back wrong. And something inside him had broken and his mouth was wide open and all his blood had poured out of him and leaked down between the cold stones, down into the fire pit. And his life-blood had killed the fire, our family fire.

21.

I Meet Long-Life

That was when Amala changed. She didn't cry or anything, she just changed. She would get up in the morning as if she too were dead already but she moved, after a fashion, and cooked something. And then she cleaned up and went to her loom to weave, but she never finished another rug. She just sat straight up there for hours and stared at the rug and then began to pick at it nervously, tearing off tiny pieces of lint here and there and throwing them onto the stones of the floor.

And the stones were why I couldn't stay— we scrubbed and scrubbed at them, all of us I think, at one time or another—but the stain of my brother's blood stayed, or I thought it stayed, and I could never sleep there again. And so after three nights without any sleep I went to Father quietly and asked him if I could go sleep in Grandmother's yurt, and he took one look at my face and nodded sadly. I put a rug down there in front of the altar and slept.

Then one day in the evening when I came in Father and Uncle were there, talking serious, and I just went and sat with them. Things had changed.

"Jampa, it's not going to work. I have orders for rugs piling up and Amala hasn't finished a single one since... since..." and then he choked.

Uncle put his arm around Father's shoulders and held him for a while, quiet.

"We'll work out something, my brother," he said in his sad calm way. "Maybe we can get one of the wives of the caravan men to handle some of them."

"No good," sighed my Father. "No good. No one knows how to weave what Amala weaves. No one knows her patterns."

That voice in me woke up just then and started to work my mouth. "I know," I said softly. "I know... all of them." And I did, from years of watching.

Uncle raised an eyebrow, and Father paused, but then he turned towards me, because I think they both knew I wouldn't say it if it wasn't true.

"I will need a little help on the technical details, stuff that any of the caravan women can show me," I began firmly, with a grateful glance towards Grandmother Tara's bed. I could almost see her perched there, with her beautiful long gray hair and steel eyes, watching me proudly as I worked her magic.

"We'll also have to set up a little shelter over there where I make the tea and take care of the cows," I went on. "But big enough for both a small loom and the big one, and warm enough when it's cold or rains."

Uncle didn't put up the least resistance this time. Father looked over towards him and he nodded. Then Father said, "Yes, all right... yes." And thus I began my Geshe studies full time.

Two thoughts were burning in my heart. I now considered the Lord of Death my formal enemy, and if there were any way to stop him, I was going to do it, with all the cruel finality he had shown to my grandmother, and my dearest brother and teacher. Secondly, I had a new idea. Amala would have her little Geshe, even if it wasn't the one she had expected. And maybe this gift would be enough to bring her back. It was all clearly impossible, but I was only ten, and I didn't know that. I also knew too much of the ancient books already to believe that anything like that could be impossible.

My first rug featured a border of one of the grand walls that went around certain cities in China. It was supposed to follow the rug around at right angles and have a lot of little intricate box-shaped corners that overlapped each other. In the end though it was a lot more like a dragon with a long strange tail that curled in figure-eights; and on top of that, the rug itself came out less of a rectangle than a crescent. I did what Grandmother would have done and used the cutting knife to make the crescent at least symmetrical, and told Father it was a new design that I wanted him to try out at the market at Kathmandu. He looked a little dubious and said he'd try, but then asked if I couldn't get on with some of the orders he'd already given me.

I told him I had an idea that I wanted to work out with some of the wives of the caravan families who were camped on the other side of the horse road, and Father was so much at his wit's end that he said okay. And I went in the afternoons and worked my heart out to learn to weave a proper rug, trading patterns for lessons. I worked well with the other women, and as the months wore on we began cooperating to produce rugs for Father. He was the unquestioned champion of bargaining for the best prices at market stalls in three different countries, and all the families were happy to have him take care of that part. I would drag home exhausted, sometimes even after dark, but my rugs improved steadily—never as carefully woven as Amala's, but with increasingly exotic designs. And there were good reasons for both.

The classes at the window were blossoming like a huge beautiful flower, and I threw all my attention into them, partly to stop thinking about Tenzing so much and partly because I was thinking about him, and hoping to learn what I could have done to stop the evil little lump. Between the milking and the tea and weaving all day long within earshot of the window, I was now catching up with my brother's classmates, and also—in the more advanced classes—hearing some of the great books they had yet to reach.

I had figured out all the special words the wisdom warriors used: basically there were four standard ways that an exchange between two warriors could go, with the attacker posing idea-scenarios and the defender normally restricted to short replies, positive or negative, which were like reaching a path that divided into two and deciding to bring the group down one or the other.

During class, Uncle would get to an exciting concept in the book he was teaching and he'd fall automatically into attacker mode, yelling out an idea to the students. Then they would bark back one of the four standard replies. To keep up with them, I would take my lunch down to the big pool at the stream—anyway it was too sad to sit with Amala silent in the dark of the family yurt. I'd find a quiet-looking cow out there drinking, and I'd practice asking questions and then responding to possible answers, depending on how her tail swished, all with the proper leaps and handclaps.

I also made up a game for when I was weaving and listening at the window. I'd thread the yarn for the next line of carpet through, and then pause until it was time to fire back the answer to Uncle's question. If it was one of the "yes" answers I would tap the line down in place with the setting stick on the left side, once or twice: *tic* or *tic plip*. Then I did the same on the right side for the "no" answers. And by the time the whole rug was done, the yes's and no's would have roughly evened each other out on either side. There in the finished rugs I saw the beauty of the way of the wisdom warriors: that by simply turning right or left along a series of questions presented in a logical progression, the warriors always arrived—in the end—at a truth which was evident to everyone present.

The new patterns that came to me poured out of my grief, and then out of my loneliness, and tiredness at night. The dream of that worst night of all was only the first, and somehow as I heard more of the ancient books my mind opened up while I slept, and memories or visions of that other country flooded through my dreams. Soon enough I realized the place had to be India, the land of the Realized Ones. And they were sweet and sacred dreams and I was happy to live in the two worlds, one at night, and one during the day.

But it was too much life to live, even in defiance of death, and the toll it was taking must have shown in my face and my work. And so it was less than a year after Tenzing I think when Uncle called me out on the stoop of my and Grandmother's yurt, for a little talk. I do remember it was Tuesday, because I remember what he said first.

"Friday, girl, I've just been to market in the village."

I stared at Uncle slack-jawed. It dawned on me suddenly that this was the very first time in all those years that he'd even been to the village, which was less than an hour away, if you walked fast. It wasn't much, Kishong, just about fifty families and a little crossroads in the middle with a few shops. But on Tuesdays a big open field out on the east side of the village came to life with the weekly market, and everyone from the whole countryside came to offer vegetables, or order a new robe, or trade a horse or cow, or just wander around to gossip and listen to somebody play a *dranen,* which was a sort of guitar we had back then.

Uncle shifted around a bit—whether with excitement or embarrassment or what I couldn't tell. He was clutching a red cloth bag up against his chest like a nervous kid with a pillow. Then finally he went on, in his very slow, very deliberate way.

"Well, you see, er... your Father and I, we've been a little worried about you, seeing how hard you're working, and never having enough sleep it seems, and... well... nobody to play with, or to talk to at night..." his voice broke, and he looked down quickly, and it was only just then when I fully realized that, of all of us, it may have been Uncle— the quiet one, the strong one—who had had the greatest hopes for Tenzing, and who had suffered the greatest loss by far. But he collected himself and looked up, with his eyes wet but his face in a big smile.

"And well, you know, it's one thing to debate with a cow, but they don't really make such good partners. Lovable, yes, in a way, but... you know... not really that *responsive,*" he mused, grinning. This time it was my turn to look down. I never could tell how many of my secrets and secret plans were at all secret from this man.

"And so we, well, we had this idea... but come, sit over here on the grass, and I can show you better."

We went and sat on the soft green grass by the path that led out to the horse road. Uncle was acting really strange, really like a kid you see, and I could feel his excitement and some of it spread to me and I realized I hadn't felt that way—well, like, fun—in over a year.

"Close your eyes now," he giggled, and I did and I heard Uncle shuffling around a bit and then he said, "Okay, open!"

And I opened my eyes and now Uncle was sitting in the grass about ten feet away and he had something in his lap—it was sort of a light tan color and at first glance I thought it was a very big mouse with long legs like stilts, and covered all over his body with this short little fuzz.

And then the puppy looked up at my face and I looked into his eyes and we both fell in love with the other at the same instant and Uncle let him go and still staring into my eyes he stepped off Uncle's lap and wobbled towards me as fast as he could; but he was still such a baby he just tipped over half way and I ran and picked him up in my arms and held him to my chest and laughed and cried at the same time.

"Oh Uncle!" I cried.

"Uh, he'll be all right, you see… just a baby, you see, still, uh, learning to walk," he explained, with a big silly smile.

My joy jumped out at Uncle and he looked at a loss for words for a moment and said, "He's a puppy, you see," and then "A boy puppy," and "Really just, you know, a baby puppy." And then the man of words ran out of words for once and just sat there and smiled with me.

You have to know that Tibetan people, we really like dogs, all kinds of dogs, from guard dogs—mastiffs big enough to knock down three or four big men at once; to terriers—little homebodies that just want to roll over and get petted on their tummies; down to the *apsos,* or the moustache-dogs, who have incredibly beautiful long hair, especially streaming down from where a moustache would be on a man. And the moustache-dogs, well, they are even smaller than terriers, really made exactly the right size to cuddle in your lap. They are as lovable to their human families as the terriers, but as fierce to an intruder as the mastiffs.

"No hair yet, just fuzz, you see," said Uncle. "But it will grow out, nearly as long as yours!" he laughed. "Just like a moustache-dog, but even better, if I do say. A real pure-bred whose parents came all the way from China, a new kind of dog—they call them *shi-tzu*. Just as pretty and just as tough, but a nice little button nose instead of the snout, and not at all as temperamental," he concluded.

"Oh, what's his name!" I asked.

"This is one name I don't have to choose," joked Uncle, looking at me ironically. "We wanted you to name him."

I looked down at the sweet little thing, who was already sucking on the end of one of my fingers, and thought—but only for a minute.

"His name will be Sering," I declared.

"Sering?" asked Uncle, "Long life? Why long life, Friday?"

I looked up at the man who was teaching me to stop the Lord of Death, and didn't know he was, and I said, "Because I am tired of death. And I want you and Father and Amala and everyone else too in the world to have a long life, to live forever and never go away."

Uncle looked at me steadily for a moment, as if he already saw the long road ahead that these thoughts would take me upon. And then he said, "Well there it is then—welcome to the family, Mr. Long-Life!"

And we sat together for a long fun time and tried to play with the tired little puppy but soon enough he had fallen asleep in my lap and Uncle had lectured me on the difference between feeding cows and feeding baby puppies; and training them not to make messes indoors; and how Uncle had found a scripture that said puppy dogs could stay in chapel yurts under special circumstances; and finally about how I should really thank Father because he had put up quite a few bags of barley (no one would ever say how many) for such a special dog, and Uncle had just been—well—sort of a delivery man, you see.

And so I made Long-Life a warm little bed next to me, and covered him at night with the nice new red woolen bag that Uncle had brought him in—which turned out to be one of those cloth slings that Tibetan women use to carry their babies. It seems that picking this bag up in the market had been a real test of Uncle's determination to help me. And before we went to sleep every night Long-Life got a long talk about what I had learned that day, just like Tenzing used to do for me near the family fire. And the baby puppy seemed to listen very carefully.

Right away too I made him a little doll to play with, and really did stuff it with some of the Calligraphy Master's scraps of paper (I got my sack re-filled whenever I went to visit with Geshe Lothar). Long-Life fell asleep with the doll in his arms the first night he got it and kept that up until he was much older—until the real trouble started, in fact; but that's later. During the day, Long-Life followed me everywhere, and helped me with everything. I never really stopped thinking about the war I had declared against sickness and the Lord of Death, but somehow with Long-Life nearby it became a more joyful war.

And he helped the whole family too. Uncle said that since we had got him so young we could teach him to do just about anything, and I dared Uncle to get the puppy to learn one of our Tibetan people's favorite little prayers, something called *Om mani padme hum.* This means "The jewel in the lotus" and is a prayer to the Angel of Kindness, a prayer that we can learn to try to make other people happy with the same enthusiasm that we show trying to make ourselves happy. And within a year Uncle had him doing it, except for the *padme* part, because Long-Life had you see teeth just like a dog and couldn't get his mouth around the *p* right.

All of Long-Life's lessons with Uncle took place out in the clearing, and one evening we all brought our dinner outside to watch, and one thing led to another and before long we'd all eat together out there around the fire and Long-Life would say his little prayer for Uncle in return for a couple of bites of someone's dinner—Uncle as a monk didn't eat an evening meal, but sat with us and had tea—and we'd all watch and laugh together. Even Amala would smile and pet Long-Life distractedly, although we could never get her to talk.

Father decided he'd do Uncle one better, which the baby brother had often done during their lives, and negotiating with special snacks he got Long-Life to stand up on his back legs and put his front paws together in front of him—in a Tibetan greeting—while he did his prayers. Then Father would yell *Bam!* (which is part of a really special prayer), and Long-Life would leap through the air and snatch whatever treat Father was offering right out of his fingers. Then he'd run around and around our circle, yelping with glee.

After a few months I took Long-Life to the big pool during lunch and sat him down on the grass and tried to practice wisdom warriors with him. The first few days, I would yell a question and he'd just run away into the sheaves of wheat and I'd have a terrible time trying to find him, because now his hair had grown out to a long light gold that matched the grain.

After that I got him to sit still for the first question, but when I jumped and swung my imaginary string of beads in the air and swooped down he was up and off again, this time so startled that he fell into the pool and I had to fish him out and brush the mud and kinks out of his hair for hours. But with time and patience, and at the expense of a good portion of my lunches, he learned to sit as still and stolid as any defender in the courtyard of the monastery. He knew he had to bark once for "yes" and twice for "no," and then we'd follow the idea down that path. I have to admit that his random replies often left me stumped for a good return.

Life settled down again, slowly. Amala didn't get better but she didn't get worse, and Father began going out on caravans again pretty steadily. When he was home, he'd spend more time over at Uncle's yurt, talking about his adventures and whatever else. I think he felt Uncle was lonely, without Tenzing. One day word came from the monastery that the Abbot had assigned Uncle a new attendant; it turned out to be Di-di-la, and we were all glad to have the kind little monk around. He'd always take the tea from the window now, and collect Uncle's lunch from Amala, and keep his teacher's yurt and the altar nice and clean—all the usual attendant jobs. Then in the early evening he'd walk back to the monastery for wisdom warriors, and to sleep.

My studies were flying along; at times now I could guess where Uncle was going with a string of ideas even before any of the boys caught it. Except that they weren't so much boys any more, and one day especially watching Drom step from the door of Uncle's yurt in the early evening (he was still always making trouble and Uncle made him stay late a lot for some kind of extra work), I realized that he almost filled the whole door. He gave me his usual smirk as though I were still the scared little girl, but I saw the man growing there in his face and paused, because I realized that Tenzing's friends were into their twenties already, and in a few years would be eligible to stand for the Geshe examinations. And then I felt again as if I had failed, because despite the window I knew I could never really be a Geshe, or even close, without being there in the real battles of the wisdom warriors—and time was running out.

Then one day I was walking up the horse road to the caravan women, to collect some new rugs for Father. I did this several times a week and often stayed for tea and talk, about new ideas for patterns or ways of weaving. And as usual Long-

Life was at my side, the long full hair of his tail sweeping down the road and then disappearing through a hedge when he chased after something.

As usual too there was a steady stream of villagers coming the other way, making the pleasant evening walk to get some fresh air, and to visit the main temple at the monastery and catch the fun of the wisdom warriors. A young woman approached me—she had a big happy face shining out through a shawl that went from her head down to her shoulders and then all the way to her waist.

She greeted me with a pleasant nod and passed by; but then Long-Life paused and ran after her barking happily, and she smiled at him too and I called him but he completely refused to come and instead followed after the girl, staring up at her, yipping with joy; and finally I had to turn around too and come after the both of them. Then she turned to me too and at that moment the shawl fell open and I saw there over her belly a red wool baby sling just like the one Uncle had given me, the one he'd brought Long-Life in. And a tiny little head covered with fuzz poked out and I giggled and thought how much the child looked like Long-Life had those first few weeks; and I looked down at my faithful dog with fondness and he looked up at me and glanced at the bag again, and I laid my hand warmly on the child's cheek to say hello and in that instant I suddenly realized how I would join the wisdom warriors.

22.

Nobody, and Everybody, Helps Me

I hadn't even put my new plan into action yet when I got help for it from two very unexpected places. I hadn't learned any new writing since Tenzing, and sometimes this made it hard to catch what was going on in the classes, since I had only the sounds of the books in my mind. And in our language there can sometimes be lots of different words that sound exactly the same; you can only tell them apart from each other once you've seen them written down, because they're spelled differently—like "too" and "to" and "two."

But then one day I came to re-fill the tea churn, and when I picked it up from the shelf my heart stopped in my chest. There underneath the churn was a little piece of paper, and for a single precious moment I thought that somehow my dear brother had returned, and that he was all well, and everything before had just been some kind of mistake.

But then I sat down and opened the paper and saw that it was not Tenzing's writing—not his careful, deliberate, elegant strokes—but rather quick and surprisingly powerful, bold brushes of the bamboo pen. And on the paper were the verses from the ancient book that Uncle was teaching Tenzing's class that day.   I ran to my and Grandmother's yurt and read them over and over, like a person who is just getting their first meal after many days without.

And then in the evening I came back to the yurt and waited quietly until I heard Di-di-la taking his leave from Uncle, and I came out on the stoop and tried to catch his eye as he passed by and down the path to the horse road. But as soon as he saw me he seemed to get all flustered, and put his head down and walked by faster.

He was almost too far for me to say it when I said it, but I finally got the courage to say it: "Oh Di-di-la."

He stopped in his tracks and came back slowly and stood a good fifteen feet away, with his head halfway down his chest it seemed, and I said,

"Thank you... it means so much to me... how did you know?"

He finally looked up and I saw then that his eyes were all sad and glistening in the sunset, and he said quietly, "I... I always watched him do it, y-y-you know. And it seemed like something that was real important t-t-to him. And so I thought it w-w-would make him happy, somehow, if I c-c-could keep it up, for him." And his voice broke, and he turned and ran down the path; and our partnership was born.

Then a few days later Father came home from a long caravan, and went over to talk to Uncle again, for a long time. And then he came out and we all had dinner together at the fire, and Long-Life played all his happy tricks, and afterwards Father asked me to come to the family yurt for a moment. It was always a struggle inside for me to go there; I wanted to help Amala and be with her even if she didn't really seem to know sometimes that I was there. But just to be near the family fire; just to see the darkened stones there on the floor; and then feel the space where Grandmother Tara had slept, looming there so empty, it was all too sad for me. I came though then, with Father.

Amala sat down, on the edge of the carpets where they slept, and stared into the fire. Father went to the altar, picked up a small cloth bag, and brought it back, and we all sat together. And then he opened it and took out a string of beads. They were Tenzing's beads, the ones with the beautiful turquoise mother-bead: the ones he had dangled over me when he played with me, when I was just a baby; the ones he had used in his battles with the wisdom warriors.

Father held them in his two palms for a moment, gazing into the deep dark wood as if it were Tenzing's face, and in the flickering light of the flames I saw how deep his pain was too. And then he pulled himself out of it, and he looked up at me, and he said, "I..." and then with a look to Amala, "We... we would like you to have these. It seems... you might be able to use them, and we... we know that your brother would have wanted that." And he put them into my hands, but what I felt was that Father—and Amala too—were giving me their blessing to finish what I had begun, for Tenzing, and for Grandmother.

And without thinking I stared at the beads in my hands and then, slowly, feeling the strength in them, wrapped them around my left wrist, as is the custom of the wisdom warriors. And I looked Father in the eye and he looked me back in the eye and he nodded, almost imperceptibly. And then I hugged him with one arm and Amala with the other and we just stayed there together, quiet, in the firelight, with each other.

When I got back to the chapel yurt I stayed up late, because I knew then that it was time to get some things ready. I went through some of Grandmother's boxes—I knew she would have wanted it, I knew she would have cheered me on even—and found some material, and got out a couple of my blouses and sewed some extra length of cuffs onto all the sleeves. Then I found a nice worn thick piece of wool material and knelt down to Long-Life, who had already been asleep for hours, and took the baby-sling covers off him and replaced them with his new blanket. I knew he wouldn't mind either.

And then I dug around again in the boxes and found a plain but beautiful long dark red shawl, and stuffed it into the baby sling. Last of all I went to the altar, and lit some butter lamps there, and put Tenzing's beads up near the little clay Angel of Wisdom. And then I held my first vigil, as I would do every night for the next three years, and I softly sang the little prayer to the Angel, the prayer that Di-di-la's name came from: the prayer that I could become a real warrior, a warrior kind and wise enough to defeat the Lord of Death, and save us all from his grasping claws.

23.

The Lady with the Baby

And so—for the next three years—if you had been the big juniper tree out along the hedge at the side of the horse road, not far from the last little tea shop, you would have seen a strange sight oh, three or four days a week. A girl, only in her early teens, but tall now, and slender, with long black hair almost down to her waist—almost very pretty, except for some kind of intensity in her eyes.

And she walks down the road from the caravan camp with a hand-woven rug rolled up under each arm, just as it's getting dark. There's this funny little dog walking beside her, not much taller than her ankles, but striding with all the dignity of a lion, with a long flowing mane to match. And they pause below your branches and the girl looks carefully up and down the road and then slips between the hedge and back behind your trunk.

And then a few minutes later a different woman, an older woman, steps back out onto the road. Her head is covered in a shawl that hides almost all her face, except for those intense eyes. And the shawl goes down on both sides, all the way to her waist, but there it falls open, and everyone can see that the proud young mother is carrying a small baby there over her belly in a sling. And villagers coming hither and thither give her the kindly nod that everyone gives to a young mother, to share somehow in the joy of the child. And she will always nod back to you but in that little way that says I'm shy and I'm grateful for your nod but please don't come up and talk to me because I really wouldn't know what to say. And the gentle young mother walks on slowly, between the little huddles of villagers who are headed to the monastery to watch the wisdom warriors fight.

On the way in the dusk my excitement would always build. I had Tenzing's beads wrapped around my wrist the way only the warriors do, but covered with the long cuffs so no one would see. Wearing them I would always feel this power streaming in to me, up my arm and to my heart, from him, as if I were carrying a mighty bow in my hand and running to war.

And this really was the feeling that came over almost anyone who approached the courtyard at that hour, as the last glow of red faded from the sky to the west, and the great brass gong atop the roof of the main temple was struck to call the warriors to battle. They would hit it once, a deep roll of thunder that burst through the walls of every room in the monastery. And then there would be a full minute of silence and then they would strike it again; and then silence, but a briefer silence. And then finally this would work up to a frenzied beating, and then one last dramatic silent moment, followed by a single thunderous stroke to match the very first one. And by this stroke the warriors were expected to be assembled in the courtyard, each sitting at his appointed place; for anyone who was even a moment late soon learned what a sting the Debate Master's own string of beads could leave upon your bare arm.

I was determined to keep all the discipline of a warrior, and so I was always at the wall by the time the last stroke of the gong had sounded. I watched the warriors streaming through the gate, heads down, no one whispering a word, brows furrowed as they went over the day's lesson one last time in their minds, and prepared their arguments. And I too would prepare my questions, the questions I could never ask out loud. But in a way this made them even more deadly.

My new baby was a perfect gentleman. I think he sensed what we were up to—as animals always do, although humans are too busy to notice—and he lay quietly upon my belly with his wonderful child-like warmth. The only trouble was sometimes when his long flowing golden locks leaked out the top of the sling—and I would get a strange look from some elderly matron nearby, and then I'd turn away and close the shawl and put everything back in order. Otherwise I kept the sides of the shawl pretty close together, so that when I was up at the wall Long-Life would poke his head out and watch too—later on I cut him some little holes to peek out of.

Over the years I concentrated on watching Tenzing's class, because I felt it was our class now. The Debate Master moved them around to different parts of the courtyard as they grew older and moved up through the ranks of the students— always closer and closer to the great pavilion, with its throne, and bench, and the Wheel of Life. Then I would move too, to a different part of the wall, avoiding the other spectators but always trying to line myself up behind the attacker. This way I could see the defender clearly, and hear both the question and the replies, and pretend I was getting in my own questions. And so really I became like the people on both sides of a chess board at once, planning my moves as well as I could but then changing instantly when the other player—or I myself—made a move I hadn't expected.

I was absorbed totally, and the hours seemed to fly by. I always took out Tenzing's rosary and held it stretched between my hands, with my elbows up on the wall and my arms free of the shawl. This way I felt more free, like it was me really clapping and shouting and leaping, more like it was me firing back the tiny powerful dart of the reply in a single word or two. The years of weaving at the window, the years of banging down the setting stick on the carpet in reply to Uncle's questions, paid off; I even found that I still kept the habit of chopping down with one hand or the other—yes or no—while I fingered the string of beads and pretended to repeat little prayers, like the other onlookers at the wall.

And I grew even as my brother's friends and rivals grew. No one could deny that Drom was awesome, the champion of the class. He stood nearly a head taller than anyone, his chest fairly bursting from his robes when he flew down the space between the rows of monks to press his attack. Stick had grown even taller, and was a quick and deadly thinker respected by all the other warriors. Hammer had grown both up and sideways, powerful and strong as a rock; he had a more deliberate but very logical and methodical style, and few defenders could keep their wits about them with the explosion of his mighty handclaps going off in their faces.

The three were all just as loyal to each other, and just as mean to the others, as ever before. It was hard for anyone to make a stand in the debates against them, especially little Di-di-la, who without Tenzing at his side often looked like a man drowning in a lake, as a debate went deeper and deeper. But even he improved steadily, before my very eyes, and anyone close to Tenzing's class could see that it would be a real fight at the end, when the young warriors stood up in front of all the other monks in their final contest at the courtyard.

On that day only a few would win the yellow hat of a Geshe, and then those few would fight again, to determine the best of the best. This was something we called *angi*—sort of like first, or second, or third place—and for the rest of his life no one would ever forget that a monk had earned it in his final battle as a student. We all felt the day approaching, a slowly-burning anxiety actually that had built up for years, and the wall didn't matter—I felt it as much as any of my brothers did. But then someone came and changed the course of all our lives.

24.

The Man with Hands of Fire

Because I was with the warriors nearly every time they met—dragging home at night with my carpets and a sleepy Long-Life trailing behind me, after a quick stop at the juniper tree—my understanding of what Uncle was teaching suddenly leaped ahead by years. A single hour of dodging and responding to ideas headed at you like a herd of angry bulls was worth weeks at Uncle's window, wonderful as it was. I found myself on the edge of understanding what really causes people to get sick, or old, or die; I found myself suddenly grasping the very secrets of life and death, and a place beyond all death, all pain— beyond all the burdens and misfortunes of life. All this had been left for us there, in the ancient books, by the ancient wise ones, for anyone else to find.

On one hand I felt like a woman walking in a huge crowd—she glances down and suddenly sees there a huge, priceless diamond, just laying there between the stones, a gift from the earth for whoever sees it first. And of course she stops and takes the gift, but at the same time she looks around, with a sort of pity and amazement, wondering how it was that everyone else passed the diamond by, and didn't get it. I often felt like this among the warriors; they knew the books, they had the knowledge, they had heard the knowledge, but I couldn't tell if they knew it, I couldn't tell if they knew what to do with it.

And on the other hand I felt as though I still needed something; as though knowing were not enough, as though—to really use what I had gained, to really help people like Tenzing and Grandmother Tara—I had to go somehow deeper than just understanding. And the answer came one day late in the afternoon, when I was almost sixteen years old, and stood there at the edge of the clearing.

I heard a strange rapping sound and came out of my and Grandmother's yurt, just as Uncle stepped suddenly out of his own doorway, throwing the flap aside in a strange kind of urgency. Uncle glared into the face of the thread sage with eyes of fire, and the lone man stopped beating his staff on the ground, and met uncle's eyes, fully, calmly.

"A traveler," he said softly, but firmly. "A traveler who seeks shelter, for a day or two, if it pleases this good house."

Uncle stared fiercely at the man, and then fiercely at the ground. You see, in our country, especially in those times, there were very few inns or other places for a traveler to stop and rest; goodness knows, there were hardly any real roads to put an inn next to, and even rough tracks like our glorious horse road turned into a sea of mud with no more than an hour's rain. So there was a code, a sacred code, throughout the entire country of Tibet: If a traveler appeared at your door, and they needed shelter for a day or two, well then you offered it to them, free, with generous meals and every hospitality you could muster, helping them in any way they asked. And Uncle had been asked, in the right way, in the ancient way; and the sage could not be refused.

"Well, yes, of course..." said Uncle with obvious difficulty, his face reddening strangely. "Our house is your house, traveler," he said, in formal reply. Then Uncle paused for a good two minutes, and finally turned and said to me, "Come, Friday," and to the stranger: "Please come, if you will." And he walked to his yurt, and entered, holding the flap open there. I gestured to the stranger that he should go first, and he did, but then as I was stepping onto the wooden stoop he turned and offered his hand to help me up, and I touched him then. And a powerful warmth, almost like a fire, came off his hand into mine—the same way that Uncle's hands always felt, but much stronger. And then something down low in my belly cracked, or shook, as if someone with huge hands had snapped their fingers there. And I blushed hard and for some reason the day I almost died came back to me.

It had happened a few years before, and I had been having one of the dreams of India, an India of thousands of years before I think. And I was stooped over a fire, and I had a beautiful ladle in my hand—bronze, with the cup carved into the shape of an open palm, and a very old worn handle of hardwood. And with it I reached into a clay pot full of *ghee*: pure butter, boiled gently into the essence of butter. And I held the ladle over the fire and said some special words and then slowly turned the little hand and poured the ghee into the fire, and the fire leapt up in beautiful golden flames, except that the flames were within my own body, deep down in my body, and the warm butter was seeping there too. And the warmth woke me up and I still felt the ghee on my belly and reached down and everything was strangely wet. And I went to the altar and lit some lamps and came back and saw everything covered with my own blood. And I knew that whatever my brother had gotten I had gotten now, even without the bump, and I was going to die.

And I laid down to die but I kept my eyes on the altar and the little clay Angel of Wisdom and kept asking him to come for me; but in the morning when I woke up I was still alive and all the blood had dried and I didn't know what to think. And I couldn't talk to Amala about it and Father was on caravan and I was afraid to speak to Uncle because it occurred to me that whatever had happened to Amala might happen to other grown-ups too if they got very sad, and really he was the last grown-up I had there with me all the time.

So finally I decided to go take some milk to Geshe Lothar, who had become my trusted confidante, and who had proved to possess a vastly greater knowledge of well just practical life-stuff than anyone I'd ever met. And I hemmed and hawed and finally came out with some of my story and he just smiled then in a fatherly way and went into a long monologue about it. And what he said was partly some very helpful information concerning women's things from some ancient scriptures; and partly just old wives' tales that I gradually figured out were all wrong; and then partly some ideas that a man who had been a monk since he was seven years old had developed about this subject all on his own over half a century, without ever being exposed to a shred of the reality of it. But in the end I gathered what he hoped I'd gather: that all the blood was something normal for a girl who was becoming a woman, and that it had something to do with making babies, and that it would happen again from time to time and I didn't need to worry about the Lord of Death showing up to get me too, at least on that account.

"Is there something wrong?" said the thread sage.

"Oh, no," I replied, and I couldn't think of anything else to say, and we came in and sat down together on the rug below the side of Uncle's bed, the chair from which he taught.

"Now Friday," said Uncle, as though he'd already made his mind up on everything. "You know that it would be very difficult to move Amala over to your yurt for a couple of nights..." I caught the drift of where he was going and glared hard at the floor, so he'd know. And he did.

"I also know that, er... well, it's probably out of the question for you to try to sleep in the family yurt..." I nodded fiercely.

"Right," he said, and stopped for a moment. "And of course I am not allowed to be in a room alone with a lady at all," he continued.

"I also, er, you know... I have the young monks coming for classes, so our friend could hardly be asked to put up with that in my yurt during the day." I glanced at the stranger, who was taking all this in impassively.

"And so," said Uncle, a lot like a wisdom warrior who had carried a little piece of logic down all the splits in the path and reached an inescapable conclusion, "I'd like to propose, Friday, that our guest stay *inside* your yurt..." he looked to me to see if I got the emphasis, and I nodded just a touch, "... during the day. And then in the evening, well, you know, as soon as Di-di-la has started back to the monastery, well then our friend can come over to my place and we'll have a nice meal and tea together, and he can sleep here.

"It means your spending all day out back here with the weaving and the tea, but I don't think that will be a problem; right, Friday?" This time it was the head of the family speaking, and of course I nodded.

I went to fight with the warriors that night but I could hardly keep my mind on it; I kept thinking about the thread sage, seeing him in my mind. He was a little older than me, but not much, I guessed—maybe three or four years. He had very long, unkempt black hair that came down over the sides of his face to his shoulders, and he wore the simple white cotton cloth and shawl of the sages, his chest bare—lean and strong, like Tenzing's had been. But it was his face that kept coming back to me: nothing at all like any face I'd ever seen. He had a foreigner's nose, but not like someone from Nepal or even India—it was narrow and strong and angled slightly like the beak of a hawk; I guessed he had to be from somewhere very far away. His skin was quite light, but his eyes were deep brown like ours. And he had a thin and somehow beautiful beard coming down his finely sculpted cheeks—it was something I'd only seen once or twice before, because Tibetan men, you see, they rarely have any hair on their face at all, and the only shaving they ever do is to pluck the occasional single hair out with special little tweezers they carry with them.

When I got home it was late but I could still see lamps going in Uncle's yurt, and hear their voices, talking. Much later Long-Life had to go out, and I saw that the lights were still burning, and I stood and watched for a while and wished I could be with the two holy men and hear their discussion—but then I just sighed over all the things that girls don't do that I still had left to do, and went back to bed.

The next morning, Amala made some nice hot flatbread and I brewed the best tea I could, and went outside Uncle's door and cleared my throat loudly (which is how we Tibetans knock on someone's door), and Uncle said "Uh-huh" loudly too (which is the way we say "Please come in"), and I brought the breakfast in on a wooden tray.

The young sage was sitting on the rug where he and I had sat the night before, and he and Uncle were chatting away now like old friends.

"So you have a monastery, and many of the sacred books, and even a place where you are copying the books to make more. It's so wonderful!" exclaimed the sage.

I set the dishes and cups of tea out and then stepped off to the side near the sage and knelt down to listen—Uncle was so engaged that he forgot to shoo me away.

"That it is!" nodded Uncle, and I realized how lonely he must sometimes be with us, without anyone around to talk to about his own discoveries in holy books, and contemplations; without anyone near him who really understood what a revolution was taking place in the spiritual lives of the Tibetan people, all due to the courage and vision and hard work of only a few—and Uncle was one of them, alone.

"And the ancient custom of the wisdom warriors—the gentle wars of ideas—has anyone been able to learn that in this land?" asked the sage.

I blushed and looked quickly at the floor, but the question was like the sweetest music to Uncle's ears.

"I think I can say," said Uncle, pulling himself up tall and straight as he sat on his bed, "that we have the best-trained wisdom warriors in this entire part of Tibet; they meet almost nightly, in a wonderful courtyard at the monastery."

"Extraordinary!" gushed the sage. "Then you must show me! You must take me! We can go together, tonight!"

Then Uncle's huge friendly smile vanished in an instant, as if someone had struck him; his eyes fell and his hands came together nervously in his lap, and he stuttered, "I... I... no, well, no, that's not possible. Impossible, really. Quite out of the question."

And the stranger's face fell and there was a long awkward silence and Uncle stared hopelessly at his hands, thinking furiously, and I felt it. It is so important to our people to keep this code, to offer our guests everything they desire, and here our poor little remnant of a family was about to fail even in this. And my heart went out to Uncle, and I said quietly, almost in a whisper, "Di-di-la?"

Uncle's face brightened instantly, and he said "Of course! My trusted attendant! A fine young man, and a worthy warrior himself! He would be the perfect guide to take you to the courtyard tonight! And then you can come back..." Suddenly Uncle stopped, frozen again. He turned to me quickly, as though we were the only ones there.

"How's he going to get back here, in the dark? He'll never find the path from the horse road."

"Di-di-la can get here blindfolded," I answered.

"No good," said Uncle. "Monastery gates will be closed long before he can get back."

A light went off in my head, but I knew I had to do everything just right, just the way Grandmother would have done. I got up slowly and brushed some stray crumbs off the tray.

"No problem," I said nonchalantly. "Di-di-la and I take him, I bring him back."

Uncle opened his mouth.

"It's all decided then," I said, smiling down at the sage, and turned and left quickly, before Uncle ever knew what hit him.

25.

A Spectre of Stone

Di-di-la and the sage and I set off as dusk gathered. Uncle came out to wish us well; he had a worried expression in his eyes and looked like there were a hundred little warnings he wanted to give me but couldn't. I bowed to him very formally in farewell, and glanced once into his eyes to tell him I would be careful, and he relaxed a touch.

Going down the horse road was completely different. Long-Life trailed further and further behind, obviously confused and put out that he wasn't getting a ride the whole way as he usually did—but I couldn't risk bringing the bag, and being recognized, or even carrying him that way in my arms. At one point the sage turned back and scooped the little lion up into his arms. "Anyone who can do all the prayers he can do shouldn't have to walk so far!" he laughed, and I knew Uncle must have been showing off our star student.

But it was the reaction of the other people on the road that had changed the most. Villagers coming out the opposite way would walk nearly up to us in the twilight, and I would raise my eyes for the usual nod to the sweet young mother, but instead the eyes on the faces opened wide all of a sudden, and then the people stopped walking, and stared, and sometimes quickly moved off to the side of the road, whispering to each other and pointing at the young sage. I felt indignant and hurt at this treatment of a kindly traveler, and walked all the closer to him, tall and proud.

The sage was obviously accustomed to people's reactions, and didn't seem to notice any of it at all. He spoke quietly but intensely with Di-di-la the whole way, asking about the wisdom warriors, and the five great books they studied, and about the monastery, and all their teachers, and lots about Uncle. At one point he even stopped there amidst the stares in the road, oblivious to the ignorance, and took Di-di-la's hand in both of his and whispered, "Such a teacher you have! You have no idea! So precious! So rare! You must serve him with all your heart, all your life!"

And Di-di-la—like all of us, who took Uncle completely for granted—seemed a little startled, and he stuttered back, "W-w-well yes! That's right! W-w-we surely will!"

And then we came to the main gates, and the sage gazed in with a look of longing at our little oasis of holy knowledge, and we continued along the outside of the high monastery wall to the courtyard of the wisdom warriors. The stares there were even worse, but I just looked straight ahead and walked on with the sage boldly, the way Grandmother would have, straight through the little clusters of villagers, parting before us like magic. We went down the low wall close to the spot where I usually stood to wage my silent battle with Tenzing's class.

"Do you know what is happening?" asked the sage quietly, obviously lost in a kind of awe as the warriors silently assembled.

"A little bit," I answered, with a smile inside me. "My grandmother explained some of it to me," I went on. "We used to come here often together."

"Used to?" said the sage, looking into my face, and it felt like he could see Grandmother and Tenzing there as clearly as if I had told him everything.

"I see," he said, before I could reply, and we turned and watched the battle begin.

And it was a wonderful battle. Our class now was tough, and smart. Like all the classes that passed through the Geshe course, it had shrunk considerably: we had lost some of our companions to sickness or even to the Lord of Death; some had simply left the monkhood completely and gone to lead a family life; others had just not been able to keep up with the grueling demands of study and memorizing and the hours of intense mental effort needed to fight with the warriors. These last were welcomed and absorbed back into the monastery without reproach, for everyone knew it was a very difficult path to tread; they would end up serving somewhere—perhaps in the temple, perhaps in the scriptorium—and they would advance their spiritual lives in those ways.

Drom, as always, was up front as soon as he could jump in. Di-di-la, as luck would have it, had "won" the toss for defender, and I looked forward to having the sage see how much he could do— even though he was surely no match for Drom. But strangely our little friend was frozen, far worse than I had seen him in many months, sometimes even forgetting where he was and gazing around the wall in our direction. Drom would fire a question and Di-di-la would just stare back with his saddest face, the big eyes all open wide and scared, his fingers nervously picking at his beads, his mouth refusing to release a single whole word at a time.

It got to a point where Drom just threw a question derisively in Di-di-la's face, and then denied him even the honor of the war: the big monk simply stood still between the rows of monks and glared at our little rabbit—no leaps, no handclaps, no yells. Little catcalls were beginning to break out in the back of the rows, when suddenly Di-di-la was saved.

The Debate Master, my dear Geshe Lothar, stepped down from his usual look-out under the great pavilion and walked slowly over to the corner where our class was seated. He came up beside Di-di-la, and changed. The big jolly monk was gone. This was some kind of spirit, a powerful spirit, towering over every warrior in the courtyard. His cloak was wrapped around him like a shroud, and he looked down upon the class gravely, with a face of solid stone. A silence fell across the courtyard.

"Who is that man?" whispered the sage urgently.

"The Debate Master, the one ultimately responsible for the education of every warrior here," and I gave the sage a strange smile.

He accepted it graciously and whispered on: "But what is he doing?"

"I have no idea," I said honestly, and stood watching that dear man and mighty spectre.

Then Geshe Lothar raised one arm silently, and his cloak followed the arm up, fanning out like the wing of some great mythical bird. He was pointing towards the pavilion.

There was a slight but audible gasp around the entire courtyard, and instantly every warrior stood up in his place, staring silently at the ground; not permitted, by custom, to look at the being that Geshe Lothar had become—and not wishing to anyway.

And then the leader of Tenzing's class—the sincere boy who I'd seen the very first day, and who already carried himself with the bearing of a future abbot—stepped quietly towards the pavilion. And behind him came Drom, and then Stick, and Hammer, and all the rest of the young men; then finally little Di-di-la, trailing behind, like Long-Life on the horse road. They gathered in the same rows before the front steps of the pavilion, and Di-di-la took his same place as defender, but with his back now to the steps, the massive frame of the pavilion centered behind him, perfectly.

And then the spectre in the cloak raised his other arm, so that now he looked as though he were about to fly up into the night itself, and a group of warriors in another corner of the square stepped in silence to the space where our class had been, and seated themselves there. And then each class stepped forward to the space left by the last, and it dawned on me what was about to happen.

I wheeled away from the wall and caught the sage by the arm. "Come now, come quickly. I must hear this." And we rushed up the wall to where the torches were brightest, pushing to the edge of the courtyard gate, through all the people around the wall and leaving a wake of angry looks and wagging heads.

The being in the cloak walked slowly around to the place where Drom was still standing, between the rows, ready to launch his attack anew. A hand came out from under the cloak and touched Drom lightly on the back of the arm, and the powerful young man dropped to the ground like a leaf, to his knees, and then sat down like a child at the side of the nearest row. And then the cloaked one moved silently down the space between the rows and stopped before Di-di-la. The boy didn't even try to raise his eyes.

And the mouth on the face of stone cracked open, and a strange powerful music came out, and it said, "My question."

Di-di-la jolted suddenly to the side, as if a snake had struck him, and then stared into the slate stone of the courtyard floor and said softly, "My honor to answer, should I be able."

The spectre stood still for it seemed several minutes. The courtyard—and all of us watching from the wall—everything and everyone, was frozen in silence.

The mouth opened again, and it sounded like how the ocean itself, the whole ocean, must sound. And it said, "Did he, or did he not, say that—after he had left us—another one would remain, as if he himself were still among us?"

Di-di-la seemed to know what to say right away, but he paused out of respect and then uttered quietly, "I cannot say, for I have not yet had the honor to study these words."

"And is that other one not still among us, even today, even in this land?"

"I cannot say, Holy One."

"And is that other one not the very code that we have sworn ourselves to live by?" demanded the spectre.

"C-c-cannot say," and I felt as though the beauty and power of it all were crushing my friend, right there.

"And cannot we say that this code that we live by has a certain essence, a certain truth, at its very heart?"

Di-di-la suddenly looked straight up into the dark sky, throwing his eyes up without letting them stop on the being before him. And all he could do was raise one hand, with its palm out, towards his inquisitor.

"And is that truth," smiled the big, hearty, jolly monk, Geshe Lothar, "is that truth not the rule, that we must never hurt a single other living creature?" And he threw his head back and laughed a mighty laugh to the sky and every warrior broke into a cheer.

"Congratulations, gentlemen!" roared my sweet Geshe Lothar, and he stepped back out of the rows, whirled around, and headed for the gate.

Tension broke from the sage in a great sigh and he beamed at me with excitement.
"What? What happened?" he implored.

"The Debate Master has just given Di-di-la's class their first words of the Fifth Book, the final book," I said in awe, and no little fear. "And so they have reached the final lessons," I whispered, "and..." I stopped despite myself.

"And what?" cried the sage.

"And six months from today they will battle one last time," I said, my voice shaking a bit. "They will battle, for the golden hat... of a Geshe."

26.

I First Hear Katrin's Name

My thoughts were interrupted by a loud "Ah, Friday!"   And there was Geshe Lothar, right across the wall from us, his hand on the gate. I blushed and gave him a big smile; he winked and looked to the sage at my side and boomed, "Well, so everyone moves up another level tonight!" And before I could ask him what he meant he was out the gate and into the crowd of villagers.

We stood and waited for Di-di-la to make his way through the throng of warriors leaving the courtyard; suddenly I was startled by a loud voice at the gate.

"Not odd at all, I'd say!" I turned and saw Hammer, right there.

"Why not?" replied Stick in an equally loud, unpleasant voice.

"Well, it figures, you see. She's just got a thing for mutts with long straggly hair!" and Hammer roared with laughter. Then Stick and Hammer turned to share the laugh with Drom but something had happened to him—I think when the spectre touched him—and he just looked at the sage and me solemnly, as if he were looking through us at something bigger. And then they were gone.

"Who are they?" asked the sage quietly. "Who was he?"

"Strange creatures," I replied heatedly, "born of the marriage of a donkey and a monkey, posing as young monks in some of my Uncle's classes. I apologize for them."

The sage smiled and looked me once up and down, and then we turned back to the wall. Di-di-la rushed up, still looking as though he had seen a ghost—which I guess he had. He asked us to wait for a few minutes, then ran to one of the heavy wooden gates in the main wall of the monastery and disappeared through it. Soon he was back with a little package wrapped in cloth. He handed it respectfully to the sage and said, "S-s-some fruit, apricots, d-d-dried apricots, you see—g-g-good for someone on a journey." And they leaned towards each other slowly and touched the top of their foreheads, which in our country is a way of asking someone special for their blessing. Then Di-di-la smiled graciously at us both and turned and ran through the gates, before they were closed for the night.

The sage didn't say a word all the way home; it was a pleasant, quiet night, just turning cool with the autumn, and the hedges of sweet-flower on the side of the road in fragrant bloom as we passed. And there was another scent, like sandalwood, mixed with their jasmine—later I realized it was coming from the sage, from the warmth of his body.

It seemed like only a few minutes and then we had reached the end of the path, and were standing before my and Grandmother's yurt. The sage gently placed the sleeping dog in my arms, and stepped back gracefully, and looked up at the moon and the stars for a moment. Then he said, "Thank you for the warriors."

I nodded shyly, and it was quiet again, and he said, "You will be back." And then he had left me, and left me wondering, and was stepping up into the waiting lights of Uncle's yurt.

The next day I saw him only when he came to take meals with Uncle; they were absorbed in discussing the details of some ancient book I hadn't heard yet. At one point I stood for a few moments with the tray close behind the sage, looking carefully at the cord that went over his shoulder and down across his chest; up close I could see that there were beautiful crimson threads woven through the white. But this day Uncle was very persistent about excusing me quickly, which of course just got me more stubborn: I brought small bowls of special tea as often as I could but was never able to hear even a whole sentence, and it riled me.

In the evening I cleaned up for Amala and went to my yurt, but I didn't feel like going to bed, and Long-Life was strangely restless too. Finally he got up and scratched at the door, and I took him out and set him on the ground, and sat on the stoop to wait. Uncle's lamps were still going strong, and the voices sounded even more animated—but I couldn't make out what they were saying.

Then I noticed that Long-Life was just standing there where I'd set him down, staring over his shoulder at me.

"Go on, you stubborn little mop! It's chilly out here!" I hugged my shoulders in my arms.

Long-Life took a few steps in the wrong direction and stopped and looked at me.

"Bushes are over there," I laughed, pointing towards the path to the horse road.

He took a few more steps the other way, and paused again; and then I realized he was headed for Uncle's yurt.

"If you need a treat, don't worry, I'll give you a little piece of Grandmother's dried cheese," I giggled. "Better than whatever you get at Uncle's, and I won't make you do any silly tricks to get it."

Long-Life just whined, the way he did when he really wanted something, and looked off to Uncle's again.

"No way," I said, more serious now. "Spy on Uncle? He'd catch us for sure, and that would be really big trouble."

Long-Life gave me one last look that was as close to a shrug as a dog could make, and headed off towards Uncle's yurt—a bushy white patch floating across the clearing in the moonlight.

"No way!" I whispered again, and took off after him. No way I was going to miss out!

We came as quiet as mice around Uncle's back corner; the flap over the window was hung up a bit on the shelf, and a sheet of golden light from the lamps angled out and down, all the way to the edge of the cattle pens. We slipped in under it, and I peeked up.

I could see Uncle's back close to the window—he was pacing back and forth there, and there was no way I could risk putting my eyes up to the crack itself. But that didn't matter; from here the voices were clear, and they were upset.

"Impossible, completely impossible," Uncle was saying.

"But you must..." the sage.

"Must? Must not!" hissed Uncle, sounding like another person altogether.

"But just..."

"Just nothing! I told you! It cannot be! The people here—people like my brother's wife, my own niece—they don't even know what I am. And they must not know."

"Is it so wrong a thing," said the sage with a kind of pain in his voice, "so wrong a thing to know the way of the sage the way you do; to know the healing; to know how to lead people beyond every sickness, to take them to their place among the angels themselves?"

"Not wrong, of course not wrong—rightness itself," returned Uncle vehemently.

"But you don't realize, you have no idea; the people around here... something happened... something bad happened. And very bad things could happen again—to my family, to my students—if people found out that I am both a monk and a thread sage. I have had to live in silence; no one can know."

"Are you saying that you don't even practice any more?" exclaimed the young man, in disbelief.

"Of course I do, I must," said Uncle sadly. "But only late in the night, very late, when there is no danger of anyone watching..." and Uncle came to the window and seemed to look down. I froze and saw the very edge of Long-Life's tail sweep across the beam of light, and pulled him to me. But Uncle saw nothing, and his back turned to us again.

"Then you will not teach me," said the sage, and I could hear the tears welling up in his eyes.

"Not that I will not," said Uncle gently. "Only that I cannot."

And then there was a long silence, broken only once or twice by a sad kind of sob, and I knew the sound well, because I had heard it in my own heart many times; many times wishing, wanting, needing to know what I had to know, to help Tenzing, to help Grandmother, to help us all, and then to be stopped from it, held back from it, denied it for some reason that was very wrong. In the length of that silence, something inside me joined with the young man. And then Uncle spoke again.

"But there may be a way, another way," he said softly, and I felt the hope rush into the sage's heart, and into my own.

"Anything," said the young man. "I will do anything. Just tell me what to do, and I will do it."

It was quiet again for a few minutes, and I could see Uncle's sad eyes searching the floor, the way he did, for his words.

"I have heard of a sage, a master sage, whose knowledge and power with the healing are far greater than my own," began Uncle.

"I doubt whether that could be," answered the sage flatly, without a trace of flattery. But I could hear the hope mingled through his words.

Uncle replied just as sincerely. "Do not doubt it; certainly I do not, although I have never met this master face to face. The sage's name is…"

and Uncle paused, and then said in a voice charged with emotion, "… his name is, Katrin."

How can I tell you what it was like, that moment? Something in my heart, like a very ripe cherry, but totally clear, like water, something in my heart burst open then, and I could feel something clear and warm begin seeping out, spreading across my chest, filling me with a kind of happiness and a kind of pain, a longing that nothing could fill. I sat there in the cold with my back against Uncle's yurt, and Long-Life at my feet, but I was like a crazy woman, and I cannot tell you if it was cold, because I felt nothing; and I do not know how long the voices went on, because I heard nothing; I cannot tell you if I even breathed, just stared, ahead, out through the sheet of gold into the dark of the fields. And then after the longest time it seems I came back, and inside my chest, and strongest at the bottom of my throat, it was just an ache, spread there. And I knew I had to try very hard to listen to what Uncle was saying.

"So first due west; just follow the sun down, until the pine forest gets thick; then angle to your left—southwest—for about a day and a half. This will bring you to what folks around here call The Rim; sheer cliffs of granite that drop a few hundred feet, and divide this tableland from the lowlands of the south.

"There's only one way down; it's where a great V-shape cuts into The Rim, worn from the granite by a large creek that descends there. So it doesn't really matter where you come out of the forest onto the granite of the cliffs—you just walk an hour or two either way and you'll see the V. Head for the point of the V and follow the edge of the creek; in some places you might have to get into the water and slide down, where the sides close in. Terribly cold but no problem if you've been regular with your channel exercises," and I could hear Uncle smiling dryly at the sage, and the young man's face set in happy resolution.

"You'll pass through some thick oak in the foothills, and then you'll know you're getting close to the lowlands; the whole way down's no more than half a day. Leave the creek as soon as you hit level territory and strike out cross-country, still southwest. It's dry and hard going for another day or so, but don't worry. You won't see the canyon until you're right up to the edge of it—drops right down into the bottom of the earth, as if you were on your way to another realm altogether. You'll find a rough path down the edge of the cliff within another half day's walk.

"Down inside, at the bottom, there's a lovely little stream that widens out as you go—it's fed from different springs that start up above and fall down the walls—quite beautiful really." I began to wonder how Uncle knew all this if he'd never been there before, but if the same thing had occurred to the young sage he wasn't saying a word, just listening hard, as if his life depended on it.

"Beautiful, but very dangerous in spots, and you have to keep your wits about you. The canyon is known for the emerald vipers—dark green, as long as a man is tall, with a poison that knows no cure, even for a sage. One brush and you'll be dead within an hour. Only the best of our kind can be with them, and you are too young to test your training yet. So careful, especially going up open ledges. Do I make myself clear?" Uncle reverted momentarily to his classroom manner.

"Yes, Elder Sage." I smiled a bit despite myself; I had never heard anyone call Uncle this before, and it felt like his real name.

"Good. And there are highwaymen: robbers and murderers, who use the canyon and its many branches as sort of a free road to travel north and south through all of lower Tibet. Only a fool would chase them down there, and they are ruthless. A thread sage they would be most annoyed at, since we own absolutely nothing and have nothing to steal, and I'm afraid they would probably just cut you up, from simple frustration. So be careful there too; agreed?"

"As my master wishes," replied the young man, again in complete sincerity.

"Now two days down the canyon you'll be getting close to Katrin,"—a pang went through my heart—"and at this point it gets really tricky. I think it better if I draw it for you."

And I heard Uncle digging around for his parchment and ink, and then there was a long silence as he drew out a map, and all I could hear was an occasional "Careful here," and "Got it!" and the like. And it was getting really cold and Long-Life was getting restless and then I heard Uncle say, "That niece of mine!" I froze. "How many cups of tea did she pour into us today! If you'll excuse me for a moment; where'd I put my boots now?"

And he was up and shuffling around near the door, and I scooped up Long-Life in a flash and ran for it, stooped over, across the clearing. His door came open just as mine was closing, quiet as can be.

27.

The Pain of Every Healer

I didn't sleep at all the whole rest of the night. I was torn between two emotions. On the one hand the name of the faraway master—Katrin—kept ringing through my mind like a bell, pealing crystal and clear, defying silence. It felt as if the wind itself were rushing through my veins instead of blood; it sang and made my heart beat all fast and there was no way it would stop or even slow for something so mundane as sleep.

But on the other hand my thoughts were troubled and confused. Many things were clear now, and I wondered why I hadn't pieced them together before: the way Uncle had crossed the fields and the big pool on the day Grandmother Tara had fallen ill; the flash of something white I'd seen across his chest that day; the way he often fell asleep at his chanting as night fell; the reason he had lived for years so close to the cattle that made noise all night, covering whatever sounds his practice—whatever it was—might make.

And then I thought of the way Uncle had stooped over Grandmother up on the ridge, and the special way he had touched her wrist, and seemed to listen to something moving inside her. It dawned on me that he knew the way of the healing, the way that sages heal, and he knew it well, if the young sage's words were true—and it felt as though they were.

When my thoughts reached this far, laying there sleepless in the dark, they went themselves then into something darker. If Uncle knew the wisdom of the monks, as he certainly did; and if he knew the healing ways of the sages as well, which now it seemed he did—if he was a holder of both of these streams of knowledge, which Geshe Lothar had told me was enough to defeat even the Lord of Death—then why hadn't Uncle healed Grandmother? Why had he left her like that, to waste away alone on her bed, covered in her own messes? And what of Tenzing? If there was such a thing as the healing, and if a person could master it, then how could it be so difficult to take away a tiny bump on someone that everyone loved so much?

And couldn't a person who knew the healing cure minds as well as bodies? Why then was this man simply ignoring Amala, leaving her in such darkness, day after day, month after month? And finally—and here I started to cry, bitterly—if there was really no healing, if it was all just books and classes and arguments and some kind of exercises or prayers that really couldn't take away a single moment of pain or sadness, then why had people given me such hope? How could they be so cruel to me, to all of us—to let us go on living in hope, to encourage us in this hope, to impress on us year after year why hope was real, how we could really do something—if there was really no hope at all, and they knew it themselves, and were in truth hopeless and helpless themselves? And so my doubts stirred to a kind of anger, and I was up before the sun, out at my fire, over towards Uncle's, burning on the inside.

It was Tuesday—market day, the monks' day off, and I knew Uncle had no classes. Di-di-la didn't come on Tuesdays either; and so once a week I'd usually take Uncle's tea and meals into him, and he'd spend a whole happy day by himself with his books and prayers. And so I made a nice tea, and some hot buttered flatbread myself, and added two small cups of fresh yogurt, and took them in to the elder and junior sages.

Uncle was sitting on his bed, as usual, poring over a rice-paper manuscript laid out in a cloth on his lap. He looked up with his sad eyes and gentle smile as I came in the door with the tray, and he watched my eyes scan the room.

"Gone," he said simply. "Gone, quite early this morning. Seems he really had to get somewhere. No matter; I don't mind a little extra breakfast on my day off, and anything left over I'm sure one of my four-legged friends can take care of," he laughed.

I stood with the tray and looked him in the eyes, such soft kind eyes, and I began to doubt my doubts, which seems to make them even stronger sometimes. And then I came to set the food down on his table but my hands were shaking and all the cups and bowls made clashing little noises, and some tea spilled out, and Uncle said, "Friday, are you all right?" and I could only look at the floor and whirl around and run to the door. And he was afraid I think to come out to me like that, and he left it, and I left it too; I threw myself into a new rug on the loom, but the doubts would not be quiet.

And then suddenly it was time to take Uncle lunch, and I went out and collected it from Amala, sad silent Amala, Amala who sat back down in the dark there even before I had reached the door. And I turned and looked at her hunched over on the side of the bed and the doubts turned to real anger, and I carried it straight to Uncle.

I fairly threw the tray down on his table—
"Your lunch, *Elder Sage,* sir"—and I tried to put hate
into the words but it was impossible to do that with
his kind face looking up at me with such pure
concern, and so I stepped back and stopped there,
standing there, and burst into sobs, covering my
face with my hands.

Uncle's face went ashen white, and he held
out his hands towards me in a hopeless way.
"Friday, Friday, I... you... you must have heard
something."

"Something!" I wailed. "Everything! You
are a healer! A master of healing! You can heal!"

He looked me straight in the eyes with those
sad eyes, and he nodded, not saying anything.

"Then tell me, now, for once, the truth! Is
there a healing? Is there a healing at all? Is it real?"
I glared back at the sad eyes.

"Yes," he said quietly. "Healing; very, very,
real."

At this I couldn't hold it any more at all and
I cried out and fell down on my knees at the edge
of his bed and looked up into his face and cried,
"Then how? Why? Grandmother Tara... and

Tenzing... why? How could you...?" and the sobbing burst out of me.

Uncle's face softened then, knowing my thoughts, and he took my hands in his warm hands and sat silent for a moment, until I was nearly quiet.

"How could I... have left them? How could I... not heal them?"

I nodded and stayed there, looking up, through the tears.

"Grandmother Tara... I could not heal," he said, quietly, and looked down sadly.

It was quiet for a time, and something occurred to me, and I said, "Was it... was it because she didn't believe in the Awakened Ones? Was it because... she worshipped those other ones, the Sky Gods, from her own country?"

Uncle smiled sadly and shook his head, slowly, softly. "No, not that, not that at all. It's all the same water, but people drink it from cups and bowls of different colors and shapes. We worship whomever our parents worshipped, really; we worship whomever people worship where we grew up. And it is no coincidence who has come to be our parents, no coincidence the place where we were born. And so we worship what we know, and it has nothing to do with that. The healing works for everyone, for every body, and for every mind, wherever they live, whomever they worship."

I looked up at him still, and asked him with my eyes, "Then... why?"

"You have to know, Friday, how the healing works. We do not heal people. We cannot heal people. People have to heal themselves. The healers must be there to show them how; be there, step by step; encourage, cajole, push, even drag; but in the end each person must heal themselves." He fell silent again.

"Your grandmother was a very, very intelligent woman," he began, gently. "And she was strong; she could do anything she set her mind to.

"And I knew her for nearly twenty years; and I know that she knew a lot, a lot about the healing even, just from talking to people—she had a very good mind, a searching mind.

"But something held her back, and I think she knew that too. She never once asked me what I knew about the healing, although she knew I probably knew. During her middle age she was just too busy with life to think of death, or of getting old; and then when she was suddenly old I think she just gave up, she just decided nothing could be done about it, because by then she had seen so many—so many friends, so many loved ones— grow old, and die.

"And so she decided that since that was all she'd ever seen, and all she'd ever heard of, then that was all there is."

Uncle paused, and gazed out to where his students would be sitting, and searched for a way to help me understand it.

"You know, there are people who can't see colors? I mean, everything to them is just black, or white, or some shade of gray inbetween the two. You know? Have you heard?"

I nodded. Father had told us about a man he'd met like that.

Uncle paused again, to collect his thoughts, to say it right. "And if you put one of them in a big, big, room by himself, and tried to tell him about red, about redness, about crimson—and he didn't believe you…"

Uncle's eyes were getting sadder. "And then you brought another man with the same problem into the room, and tried to talk to them together, but then they both don't believe, and they talk to each other and help convince each other too—There's no red. There's no such thing as red.

"And you bring another person like that, and another, and another, and soon the room is filled, and there are a thousand people there, and there are a thousand voices talking with each other, convincing each other, proving to each other, by their very numbers, that there is no red, there cannot be red; and you are crying, and crying out 'No!' and 'Crimson! Red!' but your voice is getting smaller and smaller and their own 'No!' is getting louder and louder, and it begins to drown you out..." he was shaking now, his hands trembling in mine, and his tears fell on both our hands.

"Does it," he whispered intensely at me. "Does it... does it make the red," he choked, "does it make... *crimson*... any less real? That a thousand people deny it, instead of just one? But this is how it is, Friday, this is how it is. And so people like Grandmother die, because they cannot believe anything else, because they cannot see anything else, and they have never heard of anything else; and they are too busy—or too hard inside their hearts—to ask, when they think they have heard of something else." He stopped and glared down at me through his own tears.

"So she was... she got too old?" I asked finally.

"Not too old!" His quiet voice was afire. "Never too old! *Anyone* can learn the healing! But they must want to! They must really want to! How could I teach her, laying unconscious in her own filth? How could she hear? For that is all—they only need to be able to hear; not to walk even, not even to speak! But she waited, and she thought things would be all right, or she thought things could never be all right! Even just a little would have helped her so much—and now, now..." new tears burst from his eyes, closed tight, bursting through.

Uncle's hands now were clenched into fists around mine, and I knew I should wait, and I did. And then when we were both quiet I said, "But Tenzing, Tenzing. He was your student, he came to your classes every day, he came—he listened..."

"Listened!" said Uncle in a whisper, but shouting in pain. "But did not hear! Did not want to hear! For this is the curse of youth, to be strong; to be healthy; to be bright and sharp-thinking; but not to *see*... to look around at a whole world of people who are old and feeble and who die before their very eyes and not to *see* it, not to see it coming, to believe that it will not happen to them, to believe that it cannot happen to them, to prance and skip and jump like a beautiful baby lamb being led on a string to the slaughter house. 'Oh Uncle, it's only a

small bump!' 'Oh Uncle, I am strong, I can beat it!'
And then 'Oh Uncle, what shall I do? What can I
do? Tell me what to do' only on the last day! Only
on the last day did he say it! What could I teach
him... on the... last day?" and Uncle burst into sobs
and let go my hands and turned away.

28.

It Cannot Be

We sat there both in pain for a long time. At some point I got up and took Uncle's cup to the door and threw the cold tea out on to the ground, and brought it back and filled it up anew with hot, and put it into his hands. I felt strange because just then I felt like his mother, but it felt good too. And after a while and another cup of tea I got him to take a few bites of the lunch, and he made me eat some too, and things were better.

I waited until he had glanced at his books again, and I knew he was really ready to go on, and I kneeled down and shuffled the things around on the tray a bit to set his mind at ease, and then I turned and said softly, "But Uncle, I have tried, you know I have tried. And you know I need, I must, know the healing. Perhaps... perhaps we can help Amala—perhaps there is something we can do together—and there are others, there will always be others. And so I ask you, I beg you, my Uncle, my Teacher"—he had his legs crossed on the bed, as always, and I touched my forehead softly to his feet in the ancient way, in the way of a disciple to her teacher—"please, please, teach me, teach me the rest; teach me the way of the sages, teach me what I need to know, to heal."

At this Uncle let out another little sigh of pain, and he pulled away from me strangely, and stared away at the wall.

"It cannot be," he uttered.

I was crushed, here, in the same room where I had first been crushed, the little girl clutching the little tea churn to her chest, told to leave. I stood up abruptly and grasped the tray, but his hand came out fast on mine, and held me there in the strength of that grip and strange heat of hand.

"Sit down," he said, just as strong; and then, "Please, Friday, sit down. There are things you have to know. It is time for you to know."

I looked into his face and saw it was so, and so I sat, quietly, there on the rug before him.

"It was many years ago," he began slowly, and then it poured out of him, held back for so long.

"But not that I was so young, even then. I was full, though; I had been filled, filled with the knowledge of the monks, and with the skills of the sages too, all learned in the holy land—in India at the feet of one of the greatest masters this world has ever seen. And I came home, to Tibet, as I had promised your grandfather I would do. That was my father—the grandfather you never met.

"It was hard to come, hard to come back, because of what had happened to your aunt, the aunt you never met..." he paused, and his eyes wandered off, as his thoughts did, to the past.

"My aunt!" I exclaimed. "My aunt, oh Uncle, tell me about my aunt!"

"Dakini?" he said softly, still lost in his thoughts. And then he came back, abruptly, and looked at me hard. "Oh no, no, I cannot tell you. But it was my fault, all my fault, and she was gone, and so it was hard... to come back.

"But there was the Precious One, the Abbot—not that he was an abbot then, but he was a good man, and he had been to India too, and he knew what I was, and he knew what I knew. And he was here, helping the Founding Father, helping him to start the monastery, and he knew that your grandfather had started the homestead nearby. He asked me to come, he said we would build together—that they could build the buildings, but they needed me, they needed my knowledge, to build the minds. And so I came home..." and his voice trailed off, into silence.

"It was only the first week I was back. He came from the west, nobody knew exactly where. He just walked in with nothing—no shoes, no cloak, only the thin white cloth around his waist, even in the cold. And first there was a farmer, way out past the ridge, and he'd been lame for years, and the sage—young sage, a lot like that one—" Uncle pointed to the floor next to me. "He asked to spend the night there, and the old man said yes, and they talked, they talked almost the whole night, and by morning... by morning... the farmer, he could walk again, walk strong, just like you or me..." Uncle lapsed into silence again, remembering.

"And then another house, another night, and a young girl, a very young girl, couldn't see— couldn't see from the day she was born, and then, come morning, she was cured..." another pause.

"And then the word gets around to the village, the village here, and people are pouring out to the countryside—sick people, troubled people, old people, young people, townspeople, and the monks that were here—all wanting to see, all hoping for something. And the Founding Father, and some of his friends, you see—at first they are annoyed, because everything comes to a stop: nobody to work the fields, nobody to help put up the rafters of the new temple and monks' quarters.

"And they grumble a bit and they start a few stories about the man but nothing works. And then even the sponsors—the people with the money around here, the people with the power, big traders, big land holders—they start asking about the man, they start asking the Founding Father about the man, about how he does what he does; and then, finally, there's talk about why not let him stay, why not ask him to stay, help out at the new monastery, help train the new monks.

"And the Founding Father... he feels... he feels like, I guess, he's losing his grip on things, and he and his friends start talking about sorcerers, like the sorcerers of the old days, before the way of the Awakened Ones came to Tibet, and they are warning people to be careful, and not to believe, and that the man is dangerous.

"And then finally one day word comes in— I remember it, I was standing there in the half-finished temple, talking with the Precious One, and the Founding Father was up towards the front, getting the altars put up with whatever men were left around. And they say 'The sage—the thread sage! This morning! Raised a young man from his deathbed! Said a few things in his ear and he—he just—came back!'

"And the Founding Father, he doesn't even turn around for a while, he just stands there, looking up at the half-finished wall of his temple. And then he whirls around with fury in his face like fire itself and he roars out '*Nenpa guzom*!'"

"*Nenpa guzom*: the day of the nine evil omens," I breathed. It was a day that came once or twice a year, an unlucky day to do anything important, because the stars were somehow lined up wrong; but nobody really understood except for a few fuddly old astrologers in the village, and nobody paid it that much attention.

"'Healing!' roars the Founding Father. 'Healing! Bringing a man back on the day of evil! He must be... it proves it... he must be a sorcerer!'

"And then everything moves like a whirlwind," whispered Uncle, breathless, lost in the memory of it. "And there is the Precious One, pleading for caution, and I—I'm just new, I'm just a stranger—but I can feel the wrong of it all, and I try to speak, but the Precious One touches me on the arm, and he shakes his head, and sends me back to the homestead.

"And the Founding Father... he sends word, he sends some kind of message—a horseman, all the way to Sharila, to the governor, to the garrison.

"And men ride in on horseback, lots of men—covered in dark leather, armor, spears and swords. And they ride out to the sage and a crowd is milling about confused and afraid and the Founding Father is up in front somehow, tall, evil, exploding with evil eloquence and then the people—they are afraid, they are confused—they follow, and they cry for the sage's blood, and the soldiers—they are soldiers, it is what they do—they hear, they obey, they act, they..." Uncle stopped short, fighting for breath.

Then he looked up towards the wall, without seeing anything, and whispered, "I wasn't there. Thank the Lamas of all time, I wasn't there. Your father—he wasn't any older than Tenzing was—but he was already wise, in the ways of things, and he kept me at the homestead."

And then, with anger creeping into his voice, "And the sage—he was a true sage—and he held his peace, and he *was* peace itself, and he did not fight. And they, the soldiers, first they gave him the *techak*—" Uncle stopped again, and closed his eyes. "And then, and then, *kegak*."

I looked up at him blankly, but feeling the evil even in the sounds.

"Not even words that you know," said Uncle sadly, "and it were better that you never had. They whipped the sage, and then they hanged him there, on a tree."

I shivered from the cold in Uncle's words and then it was silent again, for a long time.

"And then," he went on wearily, "and then, things settled down; and people, in time, they got busy with other things; and they finished the monastery, and they called for me to come, and begin the classes, and show them about writing, and the books, and the ways of the wisdom warriors. And I, I—you know, you could guess—I didn't really know what to do. The knowledge of the monks was very new in our country at the time; new, no, I can say it was barely alive. And in India herself bad things were happening—terrible wars, invasions—and the knowledge was in danger there as well. And even without the other half of the healing—even without the way of the sages—this knowledge is, quite simply, the most precious thing upon the face of this earth. And so I made my decision, and I agreed to come and stay at the new monastery, and I worked with all my heart, from morning to night.

"And at night I closed the door to my little room and shuttered the small window and I practiced the arts of the sages—the channel exercises, special ways of breathing, prayers, and meditations, everything that makes the healing complete. And people started to notice something, and the Precious One—who knew everything I was doing, the only one who knew—he came and warned me, warned me to be careful, warned me that one day the Founding Father would have enough of what he needed from me, and would turn on me if he knew.

"And so I became quiet, quiet as the walls of my room, and I practiced, and practiced hard, knowing that the healing was the most precious gift I could ever give to others—the way to end all sickness, to stop the process of growing old; to turn it back; and to pass untouched by the Lord of Death, on the path to the Angels themselves.

"And how many nights did I wonder—how many nights alone there did the question come: What makes us like this? How can we be like we are? How can we see a man raise another person from his deathbed, and then destroy the man, the one who could teach us to rise above death ourselves, the man who could teach us how to keep all the ones we love away from the touch of death? How could our own pride and our own thirst for people's attention and belief be stronger than the hope for life itself? And yet so we are—it is not just the Founding Father, or people who seem like him—we are all like that, we all have something of that in us," Uncle sighed heavily, and I straightened up in my seat, to give him a reason to stop; but he looked at me resolutely, determined to finish.

"No, that's not all. It doesn't end there," he sighed again.

"Then, later on, someone came to me. And they… I don't know how, they just did… they knew I was a thread sage, and they knew I could teach them the healing. And they asked me, they begged me—even as you have done today, just as you have done today—they asked me to teach them, and show them the way.

"I checked them, I examined them, as we always must. Some teachers, if they are very powerful, and if they have a connection with a person from before—from long before—they can impart the healing, and see it work, in a single night, or less. But these cases are rare beyond rare. The way that always works—the way that step by step can bring anyone to the healing—is gradual, steady, patient, sincere training; starting with the knowledge and ways of the monks, and then moving on to the special arts of the sages.

"But this person was different, and I saw it: we might come across one or two like them in a whole lifetime, not often many more than that. This one was already ready for the ways of the sages; the rest had all been prepared before—who knows how many years before. And so I agreed to teach them, for to waste such an opportunity, to waste the life-time of such a person, would be like tearing down all the temples in Tibet.

"We met at night, as is the custom of the sage tradition I was teaching to them. We worked hard and well, and it was a joy to me to have someone to grant the healing, despite all my other classes and responsibilities at the monastery.

"Yet, however much people may have noticed before, they noticed now all the more, with the two of us. And the Precious One of course came to me again with warnings, for which I was thankful, but it was clear to me what was more important.

"And then one night the Precious One comes right into my room, in the middle of a lesson, and he brings a strange message from the Founding Father himself. It says that the Founding Father knows I am a thread sage, and that I have been teaching the ways of the sages to someone, and that in fact I am teaching it this very night.

"And the message says that I must stop, and send the student away, within an hour—or suffer the consequences, despite my great value to the monastery." Uncle was almost whispering now, and gone away, gone back, no longer here with me.

"It is the kind of test that a sage is fortunate enough to receive only at special times during their training, and during their whole life. It was the kind of test that the soldiers had given to the young sage, and he had kept his peace, and I remembered. And I asked my student—I said, 'Our lives are at risk; what would you have me do?' They..." and here Uncle straightened up proudly, "they did not hesitate. They said that a few more minutes of a lesson together was more precious than anything that could possibly happen afterwards. And then I knew I had judged them well, and we went on, until the Founding Father himself came, with the men, and pounded on the door and took me away to the room, the room at the top of the temple— where the Council of Elders meets. And there they talked and decided my fate—my life as a sage, my life as a monk, even whether I would live or not." And then Uncle just came to a stop, and gazed down at me.

It came then into my mind to ask, "But your student, Uncle, your student. What did they do with them?"

"My student?" he asked distractedly, as if I were pulling him back to this room by the arm. "My student? Well, they let my student go—they sent her away.

29.

I Start for Half

"Her?" I exclaimed.

"What? Excuse me?" replied Uncle, looking a little confused.

"Her? A *woman*? Are you telling me that you, a senior monk, the senior teacher—you were teaching a woman, *alone,* in your own room in the middle of a Buddhist monastery, at night?"

"Well yes," he replied matter-of-factly, "yes, of course, alone—she was the only student I had for that subject at the time."

"No, no, Uncle," I said with exasperation. "You don't understand what I mean... I mean, well, what would people *think?"*

"Think?" he said, still looking a little blank. "Think? Why... what did *you* think, when it happened?"

"When *what* happened?" I said; now I was getting a little confused.

"When the *man* came!" he replied, with a touch of his own exasperation.

"*What* man, Uncle?" I cried.

"Why the man—the man with the claws on his hands. What did you think, when he came to get Grandmother?" and he stared me in the eyes, strong and cold, like steel.

My mind whirled for a moment, and then it stopped cold. Suddenly I saw what Uncle was saying. And he had brought me to it in the way of the wisdom warriors; he had brought me unsuspecting to a truth like a wall, and it was there, rock and solid, and I could not turn or avoid it.

Uncle looked down at me quietly, with those sad eyes—and now I was beginning to realize why they were sad. He gave me a moment to digest everything, and then he frowned and wagged his finger a bit at me.

"Friday, oh Friday, my dearest niece, Friday. Do you see how it starts? Do you see it starting there, in your own mind? Do you think there is only one thing a man and a woman can do, alone, in a room together, in the middle of the night? Do you think this is all a woman is? Has the world already taught you to think this way, at your age, so young? And will the thought not get stronger and stronger, as you get older, and then slowly you teach it to younger ones, younger women, not because you think to teach it, but because you believe it, and they sense it from you from day to day, in small talk, in small gestures? And then women, women not only wear the handcuffs, they pass them down, from generation to generation, unknowingly. Yes I was teaching a woman. Yes we were alone. Yes I knew what people would think. And I went on teaching, to try to help stop what people think... what women think, about themselves," he sighed, and stopped. It was quiet.

"Then teach me," I said simply.

Uncle looked me straight in the eyes, again. "And so they talked," he said. "They talked, for hours, the Founding Father and his lackeys. In one hour I was dead, in another hour I was disrobed, in another hour they had only given me a public whipping on the backside and disgraced our family forever.

307

"It was the Precious One who rescued me; he was afraid, afraid from the very beginning about what would happen, about what had happened to the young sage—and so he sent a man, on horseback, down the horse road, like lightning, said a man's life was at stake—told him to go to the homestead, and bring your father, and any of the caravan men that he could find.

"And Father walked into the room, not much more than a teenager really, but at that moment he looked like a giant, as if he could hold the whole world up in his own arms. And he went to work on the Founding Father—I have never seen anything like it—with his golden tongue. And by the end of the night a deal was struck, and every man in the room truly believed he had gotten the best of the deal. He saved my life; he saved more than my life—he saved my name, and the monastery, and my freedom to teach.

"And this is how it ended. I was to live at the homestead, no longer at the monastery—we would say I had come to sing the holy books to the family, and Father would assure that new holy books kept coming, and that I never finished, and that a good number of the most precious books would end up in the monastery's new library.

"I would continue to teach the young monks the ways of the monks, and of the wisdom warriors.

And there was one in particular, just a little boy then, by the name of Drom—and I would work especially hard with him, and take him all the way through the course of the Five Great Books, until the day he stood and distinguished himself at the final debates in the courtyard of the wisdom warriors—until the day he became a Geshe.

"And on that day, a prominent trader from a homestead near the horse road would sponsor a great feast and prayer in the monastery temple, to honor the new Geshe—as all new Geshes are honored—but this one as none has ever been honored before, with sizable gifts and an offering of golden coins to every monk, as well as whatever amount it would take to build a new and even greater temple.

"And finally, the hardest of all—" here Uncle looked down at the floor. "A certain monk, lately rumored to be a thread sage, would give a solemn oath that he would never again grant formal lessons in the way of the sages to any person at all—and especially to women—so long as he ever had anything to do with our monastery.

"And so you see, it cannot be," he repeated, and he was finished.

We were quiet again, for a time, and then I asked, "Then why, Uncle? Why stay here? And why stay a monk, if it means you must refuse such a thing to people?"

Uncle's sad eyes became slightly angry eyes. "Oh never think that, little Friday, and never say it again, at least in my presence. You have no idea what we are building here. Our country is like a desert, and this monastery—she is like a great lake of the purest water. People cannot live without that water. Every institution that mortal humans build has its weaknesses—goodness, monasteries are built to help the people who come to stay in them to overcome their weaknesses—but without any institutions at all, without places like this, the things that people need to know, well, they can get lost forever, instead of just misunderstood for periods at a time, which happens too with institutions.

"And what we are teaching here—the knowledge of the monks—it must stay alive, or the healing itself will die. A sage who never learns what the monks know, and who does not live by a code at least very close to theirs, will never accomplish the healing. And a monk who does not—after he has gained the knowledge of the monks—go on to practice the ways of the sages will never accomplish the healing either. They go together—goodness, they used to always *be* together, and the word was monk-sage—they go together, like the two wings that make a bird fly: must have two.

"And the life of a monk—the code of a monk: in essence, the art of never causing the tiniest harm to any living creature. If the monks' knowledge and the sages' ways are like a bird's wings, then this code is the very heart fluttering in the breast of that tiny creature. Tell me to give up being a monk—tell me to just give up the robes and go away and teach the healing to anyone I like—it would be like tearing the heart out of a tiny bird and then telling him to use his two wings and fly into the sky. I have come to the healing, and the healing itself works, only because I have followed the code of the monks, and followed it well." Uncle stopped there, breathless, and I nodded.

After a time I asked, "Do we have to be a monk, or a nun, then—to be able to master the healing?"

"Oh no," said Uncle, "I did not mean to say that. For me it is so, because it is a commitment I have already made, for my life, and I treasure it as the source of every strength I possess. But for you, for people like you—for anybody—it is only to keep that first of all codes: never to harm anyone; to treat them with all the care that you treat yourself. And to spend your whole life getting better and better at keeping this code, with every year that goes by. Then the healing can heal, heal anyone, heal anything. Defeat the Lord of Death, travel to the Angels themselves: become the Angels themselves.

"It cannot be done without the code, and—really—the code cannot be kept very well unless one has at least some understanding of the knowledge of the monks—the way of the Five Great Books."

"Then must one become a Geshe to do the healing?" I asked.

"Oh not all that much! Too much, for most people!" laughed Uncle. "No, only understand the essence of what the Geshes learn—only understand what makes all things in the world work the way they do. Only the keys—the keys of what the Geshes know."

"But a Geshe," I pushed on, trying to lead my dear Uncle to a wall of my own, an idea that was just forming in my mind. "A Geshe—surely someone who had learned so much—they would understand, surely they would understand—what is it that you need to understand, the way things work; the way the healing itself works."

"I should hope so!" exclaimed Uncle. "Especially if they were trained at our monastery!"

"And so a Geshe would make a perfect student to teach the ways of the sages!" I exclaimed. "Why, whatever had happened a long time ago, I'd say you'd probably *have* to teach them the sage's way, if they had spent all that time becoming a Geshe and had proved themselves, and really wanted to learn. Why I'd say—I'd say—you practically owed it, owed it to the *whole world*, to teach them!"

Uncle saw where I was going, or thought he did, and moved to cut me off.

"I'd say you're right, Friday. I'd say I agree with you, whatever happened in the past; and things do change, and there are ways to deal with changes without breaking one's word, which will never do either.

"But it is one thing to learn to sing a few lines, or hear a few things through a window, or read a few scraps of paper." My face reddened, and I cast my eyes to the floor.

"However noble one's intentions, " continued Uncle gently. "But it is quite another thing to stand before a thousand monks in the courtyard of the wisdom warriors, and do battle there with the best, and win the golden hat of a Geshe. You could never do all that; you could never do half of that. I tell you the truth, as I love you."

"And if I did, even… half?" I started the trap closing.

"Oh Friday! If you could go and pass a Geshe exam among the wisdom warriors—even *half* a Geshe exam!—well then I'd say the sky had turned from blue to green; and the world had flipped upside down; and yaks could pull out their own hair and weave it into beautiful rugs on that loom out there. And then, well, I'd say I wouldn't have any choice at all, and I'd *have* to teach you the healing, one way or the other." Uncle stopped and regarded me with a huge smile, and we both knew our talk was finished.

I got up slowly and stood there and tidied up the tray.

I said "Thank you, Uncle," quietly, and smiled, and went to the door.

And then I turned around there, where the little girl with the tea churn had turned around, and caught Uncle's eye and grin.

"Half," I said, snapping the trap shut.

"Excuse me?" he said, the smile suddenly faltering.

"Half," I repeated. "Half of the Geshe examination, at the courtyard of the wisdom warriors."

He nodded, slowly, unsure that he should.

"The King has spoken!" I cried, and whirled around and out the door.

30.

I Meet My Brother

"The King has spoken" is an old saying in our country. It comes from a very old story about a woman with much faith and much of the intelligence that faith gives you. She wanted to build a shrine like our little stone shrine, but much bigger: huge, one that would take say almost half an hour to walk around while singing your prayers.

But land was very expensive where she lived, and there was no hope of getting such a piece. And so she went to the King himself and asked him point-blank for that much land. And he just laughed and said, "No way." And she asked for half, and still he refused. And then she thought for a moment and asked if the King would at least grant the amount of land that would fit within the outline of a cow's skin. And he laughed again and said, "That I will do."

And then the woman, she went out and got the very biggest cow hide she could find in the market. Then she took a razor blade and sat down for a few days and carefully cut the skin into one incredibly thin, incredibly long thread of leather. And then she chose the very nicest piece of open land she could find, and walked in a huge circle, doling the thread out on to the ground. Then she went to the King to collect the deed to her new land.

And of course the King's ministers and everyone complained that she had tricked the King, but he had a strong sense of honor and I suppose a good sense of humor and said, "When the King has spoken, the King has spoken. I cannot go back on my word; the land is hers, for her shrine." And ever since then, whenever you can get someone to promise you something that they'd maybe rather not promise you but can't go back on once they have promised you, well, in Tibet people just shrug and say, "The King has spoken!"

So I felt pretty proud of myself, until I got back to my yurt and had a moment to think about it. And then I realized that Uncle was safe: it was just as impossible for a fifteen-year-old milkmaid rug weaver to stand up in the courtyard of the wisdom warriors and pass half a Geshe examination as it was to finish the whole thing. It was all simply impossible.

But then, when you think about it, lots of things are impossible—the healing itself is impossible, for that matter; I mean, how many people nowadays really believe you could heal yourself of any sickness at all, and even death, just by working on yourself yourself?   Now why impossible things like this are anything but impossible you're going to find out here later, like I did, and it's no big mystery, just certain things you have to understand and then do. But let's just say that, even at this point in my life and my secret studies at Uncle's window, I knew roughly what I could do, to do the impossible.

And so every night, late, when I was done with my singing and my writing and my thinking about the day's lesson, I would go to the altar. And there I would think about all the good things I'd tried to do that day—none of them perfect, but still good, trying to be good—and I'd go back over them carefully, just being happy that I had really tried.

And then with some special kinds of thoughts that we'll get to later I sent all the power of what I'd done ahead of me, ahead in time; I sent it to the me that I would be later, a special me—a me like an Angel that could go anywhere and help anyone. And this I did to turn myself into that me, really. The whole time I would hold my dear brother Tenzing's string of beads in my hands, repeating the prayer of the Angel of Wisdom.

318

Really it could have been any prayer, in any language, of any faith—but the important thing was how I sent the power of the good things I'd done, out and ahead, so I could really become someone that could help others. And every time my fingers reached that beautiful turquoise mother-bead I checked my heart again, to make sure I was still sending out the goodness, strong.

The last six months to the Geshe examinations flew by. I didn't miss a single night at the courtyard of the wisdom warriors. Our class had gotten even smaller and tougher, and now every battle was fought tooth and nail, knowing what was coming. I'd have my elbows up on the wall with my face to the defender, and the questions flew so fast that my hands moving right-left up-down yes-no would be exhausted by the end of the night. I'd carry Long-Life back to the tree by the side of the road totally tired but totally happy, because I knew that I really knew what I had to know, and that I'd done it the best way, the only way—with good hard work. Even Long-Life could feel the tension mounting, and there were times at the courtyard when I could hardly keep him in the little red bag, the baby sling.

I kept up my vigil and that special way of praying, every night, when I got home—no matter how tired I was. I had some idea how it could work, but no idea how it would work—I just kept it up, with patience and a good heart, up to the very last day before our class was to join our final battle.

That day before—I will never forget it, for again it was one of those days that changes everything. Uncle had canceled all his other lessons and spent the whole morning with our class, going through a few final debates; trying to inspire the young men to do well and be good, especially to each other; and attempting to calm down everyone's case of nerves, although to tell you the truth Uncle seemed more nervous than anyone else. Imagine! All his years of effort coming to fruit with these, all of them, his pride and joy. And—as he and I both knew now—the approaching end of one big part of the deal that Father had struck with the Founding Father.

The young men filed out of Uncle's and stopped in a little huddle, there at his front step. They were comparing precious little slips of paper that they'd drawn out of a special silver urn atop the altars of the main temple at the monastery, just that morning, very early, at the start of the first of the daily prayers there.

The papers gave the subject to be debated by each pair of warriors: your opponent was the only other monk who had pulled the same subject. The first day of battle was always held on the first day that the moon began to appear again, just a sliver—since this was considered good for beginnings. One would attack, and one defend. Then a week later—on the half moon, also an auspicious day—the two would meet again, switching the two roles. The subject you pulled on your paper, and your opponent, were crucial in how your performance looked to the Abbot, who would be the judge of the contest.

"Ho!" exclaimed Stick, glancing around at the slips. "So we finally get to prove that a quick Stick to the head can beat a big but *very slow* Hammer!"

Hammer turned and grinned at him, obviously very nervous, but managed to say, "Sticks are born of trees," meaning things that didn't move very fast at all.

And then I saw Di-di-la's face, and it was pure anguish, on top of the kind of nervousness that's so bad you can walk around half a day and not hear a single thing around you. And I looked at Drom, clutching his own little slip of paper, looking at Di-di-la with a kind of terrible glee, like a huge powerful snake that has cornered an innocent little bunny. I knew what had happened, and Long-Life and I marched over to save the day.

"Di-di-la! Isn't it exciting! Just tomorrow and the whole thing starts! Which subject did you draw? Who's your opponent?"

Di-di-la's mouth jerked here and there a few times but refused to open. Finally he just raised his hand, still clutching the paper, trembling like a leaf, and gestured towards Drom. Drom smiled widely; Stick and Hammer snorted.

"Well, too bad for Drom! I'm sure he'll be standing there by the end hopeless, without a single word to say!" I smiled, or at least gave it a good try.

"Oh yah! I'm sure!" exclaimed Hammer. *"Ki kup ne nima shar yong!"* he shouted, pointing down to Long-Life, and then the terrible trio was off past my yurt on the path to the horse road, roaring with laughter, slapping each other on the back.

My face got very red, I think, and even mild-mannered Di-di-la's jaw clenched with anger. Because, you see, what Hammer said means "Oh sure, and the sun is going to rise tomorrow out of a dog's rear end." This is an old way in our language to say that something is just 100% totally impossible. And I think what made Di-di-la and I both upset was that we knew it was true: there was no way Di-di-la could ever beat Drom.

It was quiet for a while and all the students were well gone, when Di-di-la suddenly frowned and looked down at the ground, and then finally said to me, "Friday, there's s-s-something I have to ask you. S-s-something important."

"What's that?" I said, trying to sound cheerful.

"There's s-s-something I n-n-need to know."

"What?" I said, suddenly feeling a little alarmed by the tone of his voice.

"I n-n-need to know, whether you are p-p-planning to come to the debate tomorrow—to the final battle, our Geshe examination."

I smiled ruefully. Come, yes. Battle, no. But I just said, "I wouldn't miss it for anything. Even Uncle is going to come. He said we could go together."

"Uh... oh... I see," stumbled Di-di-la. "But that's not who I meant; I mean, that's not the you I meant; I mean..."

I let out a little laugh. "Di-di-la, what are you trying to say? Is there some other me running around that I don't know about?"

This time it was Di-di-la who got all red. "Er...well... I mean, Friday, what I mean is... is well, do you know if... if the l-l-lady with the *b-b-baby* is planning to come?"

My heart stopped cold. I glanced over my shoulder at Uncle's door, still open, and then looked Di-di-la in the eye. "I think," I said, "I think maybe we could talk about this over near the path, near my yurt—much more shade there, you know," I said, raising my eyebrows and pointing with my head.

Di-di-la glanced at the door and nodded. "Oh yes, of c-c-course, I see..." he said, and we walked across the clearing, around the corner of the yurt.

"Di-di-la!!" I hissed. "How... how on earth... how did you know?"

He smiled widely and glanced down at the ground again, shyly. "Well, Friday, you know, first of all..." he looked around a bit with those big scared eyes, searching for the most diplomatic way to say it. "Well, first of all, you know, it's kind of weird for a lady to carry the same baby in the same bag for three years straight, and the baby never even grows an inch—for three years, the same size—just about the size of a lapdog, actually," and he grinned and looked down at Long-Life, who was staring up and listening attentively. Long-Life wagged his luxurious tail a few times at Di-di-la, as if enjoying the joke.

"Oh," I said, reddening again. All this time debating logic, and it had never occurred to me that my baby should have been growing. I couldn't believe no one else had noticed it.

"But that's not how... how I knew, at the very beginning," he said quietly. He looked off to the horizon for a long time and then came back.

"It, it was the b-b-beads," he said. "The beads in your hands, when you put your elbows up on the wall and start making answers with your hands, like you do with the setting stick when you weave."

Did I have no secrets? I wondered. But out loud I just said, softly, "Tenzing's beads."

"I know," said Di-di-la, with a kind of reverence, and sadness. "Because, you see, the mother-bead, the piece of turquoise—it was mine, I got it from my grandfather when he passed away—and I... I gave it to Tenzing, when we were just little kids... on the day, on the day that we..." he stopped for a moment and began to weep. "On the day that we became blood brothers," he whispered, and turned around so I wouldn't see him cry.

I touched him softly on the arm and left him alone with it for a while. "So we're family," I said then, and he turned around and nodded with a grateful smile, and then in a moment he could go on.

"And so those beads—I'd know them anywhere; the turquoise caught my eye right away, and then in a day or two I'd figured out what you were doing, and how your hands moved. And then, I... I..." he stumbled again, to a stop.

"You what?" I said gently.

"I... oh Friday, don't you know? Three years! For three years I've been watching your hands, every time it was my turn to be the defender, and I've been following you—I've been speaking for you; and you've been thinking for me, for *three whole years!*"

I stared into Di-di-la's face with astonishment, trying to grasp what he'd just said. But then the words were pouring out of his mouth.

"And tomorrow, you see, the final day—the day that I and all the others have worked for our whole lives—tomorrow, I'm the *defender!* Against *Drom*, the very best warrior in our whole class!"

I stared at him, still not grasping it.

"Friday!" he was nearly yelling at me now. "Friday! Don't you see? Don't you get it? If the lady with the baby… if she doesn't show up at the wall tomorrow evening… well then, I'm dead! I'm totally dead!"

I held my hand up for a moment and shook my head clear, and then glared into Di-di-la's even wider eyes.

"Di-di-la," I said, my voice shaking. "Do you mean to tell me that for… for three whole years… you've just been giving my answers every time you're the defender?"

He nodded, fast at first, and then looking at the ground, ashamed.

"But what have you been doing when you have to play the attacker? That's no simple yes or no!"

"Oh that," he mumbled. "That, being the attacker, I just muddle through, you see. It's not that I don't get Uncle's lessons; I do, and I love them, I love everything, and I see how—with what he is teaching us—we can come to help everyone there is.

"But it's the warrior thing, you see—I get nervous, I just freeze all up, inside. When I'm sitting on the stone there and somebody is standing up in front of me—especially somebody like Drom—and they're leaping here and there and slapping their hands in my face and screaming some question at me well I just go blank, I go totally blank. And even when I don't go blank my m-m-mouth, my m-m-mouth, it gets all tight and twisted up, you see, and even if I can think the words they don't come out.

"But then I found that when I look at your hands move—when I think of you helping me, and Tenzing helping me, from his own beads right there in your hands—then I see the answer in your hands, and I understand it, and I know why it's right and I don't feel scared, and I can say it.

"But by myself... by myself... without my sister," he smiled at me, "I'm a dead Di-di!"

I nodded and looked down at the ground in thought, and there was Long-Life staring up at me with that cute button nose and his funny pink little tongue. He caught my eye and glanced over at Di-di-la and then back at me and threw the long silken hairs of his tail up in the air and down hard on the ground, like a warrior's handclap—and in that instant I saw half of a Geshe examination delivered into the palms of my hands, on the last possible day.

"Di-di-la, my dear brother," I began, with quiet excitement. "Girls don't do this, not usually, but I have an idea…"

31.

Something Girls Do

The next morning I got up and made the family tea—I took some to Amala, who was just the same, sitting in the dark, and sat with her for a while. I thought that she must have sensed what was going on, that this was the day her little Geshe would have stood for his final exam, but she didn't show a thing. I sighed and went and took Uncle his little churn.

"Friday! Excellent! Not too much, got to sit for hours in that crowd today! Are you all ready to go?" he exclaimed.

"Uncle, we still have about eight hours to get ready," I smiled. He was as excited and nervous as a little boy.

"Oh really?" he said, in disbelief, looking out the door to the morning sun. "Oh yes, yes, does seem that way, come to think of it.

"Everything's taken care of," he said, in exuberation. "A couple of your weavers from the caravan camp are coming over in the afternoon to stay with Amala until we get back. And I must say, Friday, that you have really done something wonderful with them, all those nights over there working so hard. Before he left on this last trip, your father told me that all their carpets are as fine as the ones Amala used to make, and that the families are very grateful for the extra income they get, especially when your father does the bargaining for them in the market. It's helped everyone a lot, and you should be proud."

It was a day for the fruits of good hard work, and I smiled at Uncle and thanked him. Then I leaned over to pour the tea and suddenly straightened up in pain.

"Oh!" I said, clutching my tummy.

"Something wrong, child?" asked Uncle, with concern.

I stood there and took a few deep breaths and managed a grimace.

"Oh nothing Uncle... just... just you know, something girls do; that time of the month."

I looked about a bit in distraction and said, "I'm sure it will pass—maybe though I'll just go and, you know, lie down for a bit."

Uncle nodded and appraised me with an understanding look. "Yes, yes, by all means. Get some rest. You deserve it."

And so I spent a few hours lying down in my yurt with a bored Long-Life looking at me with curiosity, and went through possible debate scenarios, waving my hands around now in earnest, because I knew that every gesture today would have to be precise. Poor Di-di-la had not only drawn the most ferocious opponent, but the subject he was supposed to debate was also one of the most difficult in the entire Geshe course: the study of how the mind reasons things out, and how it is that we can perceive and recognize the things around us.

At noon I went over and took Uncle a pretty large lunch, as it would be a long walk and an even longer ceremony. I made sure to hold my tummy the whole time, and he finally sent me back to my yurt. I laid down and practiced and started to get an increasingly bad case of nerves, and then suddenly Uncle was tapping on my door, saying it was time to go.

"Oh, Uncle," I moaned, "I don't know if I can make it."

He came inside and stood there at the door gazing down at me; Long-Life was a really good boy and glanced up at Uncle with big doleful eyes, to match the mood. Uncle looked magnificent, with a new set of rich red wool robes, and his golden ceremonial cloak folded over his shoulder. He had his old warrior's beads wrapped around one wrist, and with one finger of his other hand he held a small brass ring. This was sewn to a golden string that went up to his shoulder, tied there to the end of his golden Geshe hat. It was very, very old, and of a very old design from India; Uncle, being a very modest man, wore it only when he was really expected to, at ceremonies and such.

Geshe hats though are so tall and pointy that they fall off at the slightest excuse, and so the monks usually tied a string on the bottom of them and flopped them over their shoulder and carried them like that, holding on to the string, until they got to wherever it was that they were actually supposed to sit down and put the thing on their head.

"Really bad, huh?" said Uncle sympathetically.

"Oh yes, I'm afraid so," I groaned. "And on such a day! I can't believe it!"

"Yes!" said Uncle, thoughtfully. "On today, of all days! And I can hardly remember the last time you've been this sick! Better let me check!" And before I could say a word he had my wrist up in his toasty-warm hands, fingers spread out on some kind of subtle little streams of energy flowing beneath the skin.

Uncle was quiet for a minute or two and then got up. "Hmm," he said. "Perhaps... perhaps you need to rest... a little more?"

I nodded glumly. Uncle always knew too much, and never said enough.

"I see," he said, with a slight grin. "Well, guess I'll have to run along without you..."

I nodded again.

"If you need anything, just go over to the family yurt and tell one of the ladies who's helping Amala," he said, with something like a serious tone.

I nodded again, smiling weakly. He went out the door and then popped his head back in and added, "By the way—don't worry about any tea in the morning. I'll be up and gone to the monastery bright and early—some kind of meeting with visitors from out of town. Should be back by noon, I hope," and he was gone.

I waited as long as I could for Uncle to get a good head start. Then when I figured I had enough time to make it to the courtyard I got the baby sling out, rolled up one of Grandmother's rugs and tucked it under my arm, and went and told the caravan ladies I really had to get it over to the camp. Then my baby and I took off as fast as we could go, changing into the shawl and the sling at the tree near the road.

I had never seen so many people in my whole life; a giant milling crowd of monks and villagers was backed up all the way out the front of the main gate of the monastery, trying to push their way past to the courtyard. I looked at the crowd and then at the late afternoon sun, and knew we would never make it to the wall in time. And so I just set off in the opposite direction, straight across the empty winter fields, to come around the back way. This meant circling the entire monastery wall, and we came out at the back of the great pavilion just as a magnificent spectacle was starting to unfold.

The entire pavilion, and every inch of the floor of the courtyard, was covered in a sea of golden ceremonial robes. Almost every monk wore a Geshe hat; the monastery kept a huge supply on hand for special occasions, and on days like this they were handed out, and everyone got to dress up: sort of good luck for those who would never be a real Geshe, just to wear the hat every once in a while.

And there was a mighty chant rising up into the air, the hats swaying like a giant field of golden wheat, swinging left and right in unison, with the rhythm of great drums and cymbals and the piercing echo of horns carved from priceless white conch shells.

There was a wide aisle left open between the rows of seated monks; it went all the way from the courtyard gate to the steps of the great pavilion. A procession was flowing out of one of the gates in the monastery's main wall, and making its way up the aisle. In the very front were two stout young monks with very red, very chubby faces, blowing with all their might on ceremonial trumpets. In counterpoint to their blasts came the deep bass roar of the great trumpets, almost fifteen feet long, supported on special wooden stands atop the roof of the main temple. And between their song flowed huge waves of sound from a great gong, nearly six feet across, also set on the temple roof. And so the sounds and the colors fairly struck against Long-Life and I, like a strong wind, as we stood at the back wall and watched the high Lamas make their entrance.

First came the Debate Master, my dear Geshe Lothar. He wore the great cloak of his office, and it made his already sizable bulk look as big as three ordinary monks, a great block of red working its way slowly to the pavilion. Behind him came the Precious One, the Abbot, with a handful of attendants. He looked as bright and cheerful as ever, with an extra sort of light beaming from his face—the joy I think of seeing all their hard work with the young monks come to this wonderful conclusion.

And then came the Founding Father, with a very special Geshe hat, incredibly high, so that he towered over the entire procession. His chin was cocked towards the sky, and he surveyed the mass of people with a cold air of pridefulness; I sensed that he was eagerly anticipating the glorious slaughter that was about to take place as his nephew made short work of the hapless Di-di-la.

Clutching the arm of the Founding Father, and supported on the other side by several watchful attendants, walked a very, very old Lama whom I had never seen before. He wore a kindly smile on his ancient face, but it was set in a painful way, and he was obviously having trouble walking so far through the throng.

I glanced at the opposite wall, the one where I would have to stand if Di-di-la were to see my answers, my hands. I breathed a sigh of relief; thankfully, there were very few people there, just some piles of timbers stacked not far from the wall, and nearly as high. I knew I could make my way around in plenty of time, and so I stood and took in the sight or the entrance of the two warriors.

They walked side by side, slowly, in through the gate. Drom cut an awesome figure, his huge shoulders draped in new ceremonial robes of golden silk, and a Geshe hat atop his head that looked as if it had been there the day he was born. Di-di-la at his side looked like a small child out for a walk with his father: his eyes were open wider and more scared than I could ever have imagined possible, and the end of one of the countless piles of ritual robes wrapped around him had come loose and was trailing behind on the ground, unnoticed only by Di-di-la. His Geshe hat kept tipping over one way, and then the other, so that actually he was attempting to stride down the aisle gracefully with both hands up on his hat.

They made their way to the front, up the steps of the great pavilion, and sat down side by side on the bench there, facing the huge crowd. Off to each side, up on the pavilion floor, I could see our classmates, who would each be taking their turn in the coming days. Stick was sitting tall up near the examination bench, and Hammer's broad back showed in the last row, at the edge of the pavilion stage. Geshe Lothar made his way through them and took up his place as the Debate Master, always standing, right behind the two young warriors.

The high Lamas had already each climbed the steps to the top of their thrones. These were little platforms up higher than Geshe Lothar's head and were set well back behind the examination bench, shaded from the afternoon sun by the roof of the great pavilion. The Precious One occupied the middle throne, with the Founding Father on the throne to his left and the Ancient One to his right. This meant that the old Lama was senior even to the Founding Father, and I had never heard of such a thing. I turned to a monk who stood nearby, setting torches up on the wall for lighting later on.

"Venerable One, if you please," I asked. "Can you tell me who that older Lama may be?"

"Ah," he said. "A visitor, and a welcome one; perhaps the greatest wisdom warrior there ever was. His name is Kachen Supa, and he is the High Abbot of the great monastery of Delek Rirab, many days' ride to the east of here. He is to be one of the judges."

"*Judges?*" I exclaimed. "But I thought... I thought... isn't it the custom for the Precious One to serve as the judge, the only judge?"

"Usually goes that way," replied the monk, with a little smirk. "But seems like the Founding Father, he decided he would be a judge too, and — you know — he usually gets his way around here."

I groaned inside. The Founding Father wasn't leaving anything to chance. Even if by some miracle Di-di-la beat Drom, he would still lose.

"And the Precious One," continued the monk, "he did — as he always does — a little side-step to, you know, to sort of even things out; and well my guess is that he talked the Ancient One into coming to be a judge too, and not even the Founding Father could refuse us an honor like that. And so here he is, along with a good hundred young warriors newly trained at their own fine courtyard. Why, here they come now!"

And we looked to the gate in the main wall and there was a great stream of monks pouring out, dressed in maroon-colored cloaks, every one, stepping forth three-by-three in a quiet dignity. It occurred to me that there was no place they could possibly squeeze in to sit; and then in the next moment they had veered off to the right, and were beginning to assemble in rows atop the timbers. And suddenly I realized why the timbers were there, and suddenly I realized why the opposite wall had been free, and then with a sinking feeling I realized that I would never be able to get to the wall in front of poor Di-di-la.

32.

The Warrior Arrives

I froze then for a few minutes and watched the disaster begin. The chanting and the horns and cymbals and the noise of the crowd of spectators vanished, all in an instant, and the entire scene before me was nothing but expectant silence and the extraordinary beauty of sparkling colors and devout faces.

Drom rose slowly in the total silence, with a mighty look of sheer determination on his face, and took about ten solemn strides out away from the examination bench, towards the crowd. This left the terrified Di-di-la sitting alone to one side of the seat, looking as though he might jump up and run away. Even from where I was I could see Di-di-la's head turning from side to side, desperately scanning the immense mass of people that had closed in upon the wall, on each side of the timber platform. I waited in agony for the call to battle, the first word of wisdom, from the Mother Tongue: the sound of *Di!* And as soon as it came, I knew, it would be too late to help my brother.

Drom slowly removed his Geshe hat, handed it to one of the attendants nearby, and then turned grimly to face his victim. One powerful arm came out from under the rich ceremonial robes, and with practiced dignity he removed the corner of his upper robe from one shoulder: a salute to his opponent, however unworthy. Di-di-la nodded back, as is the custom, and in that moment I saw his head stop moving from side to side, and his gaze closed bravely on Drom's eyes. Whatever had happened to his savior with the baby, Di-di-la was going to take his defeat like a true warrior.

Then the most extraordinary thing happened. Drom raised his face to the shining sun and the crystal blue sky overhead and roared *Di!* And in that same instant he was hurtling towards Di-di-la, bursting through mid-air. Di-di-la flinched and ducked his head, and in that single graceful leap Drom swept down with one arm, snatched the Geshe hat off Di-di-la's head, and— still in flight—kicked off the top of the bench with one foot, spinning around in the air and landing not far from where he had started. He threw up his arm with the hat clutched in his mighty fist and roared out again *Di!* at the top of his lungs.

Suddenly the crowd woke up. It is a custom in the great examinations for the monks looking on to join in the intense excitement, to cry out their approval or disapproval of whatever the warriors have said in that moment. And so a great murmur of astonishment swept through the crowd, mingled with a low rumble of disapproval, for this was nearly taking the traditional hazing too far. I saw a few of the older monks, the ones in front—and I knew Uncle would be there somewhere—begin to wag their heads.

But then suddenly Drom was standing right in front of Di-di-la, towering over him. Drom set the hat across both his palms, and in an ancient gesture of respect bowed, and offered forth his hands with the hat. A loud gasp of approval, and relief, and then amusement broke out from the entire crowd. When Drom straightened up again I saw him glance slightly towards the Founding Father. There was an almost imperceptible nod of approval, and I guessed who had planned this opening attack.

Di-di-la finally looked up, sheepishly, and with shaking fingers plucked the hat away. He tried to set it back on his head, but the tactic had worked perfectly: he was so rattled that there was no way he could keep it on. And so he just took it off and set it to the side, on the bench, and looked up with resignation to meet his doom.

And Drom was ready to give it to him. The first questions flared from his mouth like arrows afire, and Di-di-la's face went white; his mouth was working open and shut in sort of a spasm, without a single word coming out. And when I saw this my heart broke, and the warrior came out in me, for the first time really.

I whirled from the wall and threw myself into the mass of bodies jammed against me now on every side, screaming like a mad woman.

"The baby! Oh, my baby! He'll be crushed!" I clutched the red bag with Long-Life up against my chest. "Oh let me through! Please, let me through!"

When they had time, the startled people parted before me, like magic; and if they were too slow they were shoved to the side, or I flew around them, or got down in the dirt on my hands and knees and clawed through the forest of legs with brute force, still screaming "The baby! Oh, my baby!"

And the sun was beating down from the cloudless sky, and I was covered in sweat, with dust smeared over my cheeks and tears of rage flowing down through the dirt. I glanced across at Di-di-la; he was taking a real beating. His mouth was working again and he was wailing out answers, in an almost incoherent anguish, but just "yes" or "no" at total random. Drom wasn't giving the least quarter, the least mercy. He drilled the questions and when the pitiful answers returned he stood and stared with a frank look of disdain, turning to the crowd and raising his palms to the sky as if to say, "How did this fool ever make it this far?"

And at first there were catcalls, and then louder and louder boo's, and then the worst of all — the thing that pricked the rage in my heart — a thousand monks settling down into bored but polite silence, then turning to talk to each other about what kind of refreshments might be served, or whether tomorrow's pair of warriors might be something of more interest. And I looked away again and fought my way screaming down the length of the wall, towards the gateway of the courtyard.

33.

Help From the Sky

"Can't come this way, ma'am." I looked up from my struggle and saw three cherubic-looking young novices blocking my way down the wall. Behind them there was a sea of red robes spreading out against the wall—all novices, the kind that get stuck with kitchen duty. In their midst I spotted the soot-streaked face of the Master Cook, shouting out directions, with stacks of wooden tea churns forming everywhere around him on the ground. Refreshments for the crowd, I realized, and nowhere to go, not even down. I looked over towards the battle, or rather slaughter, and saw that I was still too far from the front for Di-di la to see me.

I put my hand on the wall and stood up tall there—did I tell you I had just about grown up?— on my tiptoes. On the other side of the small army of kitchen helpers I could see the courtyard gate—

still a little far off to the side of Di-di-la's line of sight, but it just might work.

The kitchen monks had cleared that whole area of villagers, but there standing head and shoulders over all the red shawls was a single farmer—a huge red-faced man with his hand resting on the gate-post, watching the warriors with a scowl that said, "All the trouble it took me to get this spot, no way I'm moving." And in fact no one was even asking him to move. To me he looked like heaven: my one last hope, if I could only reach him.

I turned away from the wall and pushed through the people, circling around the monks, still screaming about the baby with my head thrown back and tears and dirt all over my face. When I got to the line of novices still pouring out of the monastery doorway with tea churns I just ducked down under Grandmother's red shawl and turned into their line, flowing with them back towards the courtyard wall. In a minute then I was near the gate, standing at the side of the huge farmer.

I tapped him on the elbow, which was almost as high as my head; the scowl turned my way and glared down. I held up the baby sling and the face broke into a kindly grin.

"His uncle!" I yelled, over the noise of the war and the clumps of bored conversation.

"'Scuse me?" said the big man.

"His uncle!" I repeated. "His uncle! That's his uncle up there debating today! Oh he has to see it!" I pointed to my baby. "Once in a lifetime thing, you know!"

"Oh, right!" the man yelled, and he stepped gallantly back from the wall about a foot—crushing three or four young cook's assistants in the process.

"Which one is he?" shouted my hero, as Long-Life and I slid up against the wall.

I threw a grateful, demure smile back over my shoulder. "The winner, of course," I shouted back, and turned to make my war.

I stood again as tall as I could and tried to catch Di-di-la's eye. But he was just staring out towards Drom like a mouse caught by a cat in a corner, hypnotized by his approaching demise. I shouted two or three times but it was no good; people had spotted the tea churns, and the great debate was about to deteriorate into a raucous tea party, while Drom went on clubbing the corpse at his feet.

I waved my arms but Di-di-la simply wasn't looking. I started to cry again, and put my arms down on the wall and stared at them. Then it was all quiet again, but this time it was the silence, the one that came to me alone. I looked at Tenzing's beautiful beads, wrapped around my left wrist. I felt the coldness of the wall, the stone, beneath the growing shadows. I looked about me in the silence and saw more young monks pushing torch sticks into their holes on the wall. I looked over at the hundred glorious warriors from afar and saw the last shaft of golden sunlight creeping up through their ranks, as the sun finally touched the roof of the great pavilion.

I looked up at the last of the deep blue of the sky and the thought came to me, "I wonder what Grandmother would do right now, if she were here?"

And then I heard a woman next to me, and she said, "Hold up the beads."

I looked around, still in silence, but there were only men there, all men: the big man, and the monks.

And so silently I raised the beads, in my left hand, and held them there in front of my heart.

"Higher," the voice came again. "Higher, as high as you can reach."

And still in silence I held up the beads, all the way up, thrusting them into the blue sky. And they sank into that last shaft of golden light, and I looked up to the top of the great pavilion, and there was the sun lying upon it like a great golden egg, and in the center of the egg there was a shape like a woman, as though she herself were sitting there, on the very peak of the pavilion roof, as she had on the throne in the main temple, so long ago.

And then I looked ahead at Di-di-la and saw bright blue patches of light dancing across his face. He squinted and looked up in the same moment that I did, and together we saw the golden light throwing itself across the turquoise mother-bead, then splashing back in brilliant rays of blue. And Di-di-la watched the pureness of the blue like that, for a few long moments, and then his eyes and mine came down too at the same moment, and welcomed each other.

"This one's for you, Tara... Grandmother... Tara," I smiled, and raised the great sword of those two little weaver's hands.

34.

War is Waged

"When you want to prove something to somebody—when you want to show them an idea that they haven't thought of yet—you must use a reason, correct?" Drom was saying, using very simple words now, a kind of taunt to remind Di-di-la of how hopeless the situation was.

But Di-di-la had already begun the change. He looked down calmly at his Geshe hat lying on the bench, and picked it up. He put it on slowly and made a fuss of adjusting it, which gave him an excuse to look over to the side and see what my hands were saying.

Left hand up, once: "C-c-correct," Di-di-la replied.

"That's *good!*" taunted Drom again. "And a reason can be defined then as something which proves what you are trying to prove, correct?"

Di-di-la touched his fingers to his forehead, as if to give it a thought, and glanced under them to the side, to my hands.

Right hand up, once. "Not so?" said Di-di-la softly. Drom looked startled and called out, "What did you say?"

I nodded up and down, a big exaggerated nod. "Not so!" repeated Di-di-la, trying to sound sure of himself.

Drom took a step backwards and corrected himself in an instant. "Or can we say, rather, that a reason can be defined as something that proves, in *three different ways*, what you are trying to prove?"

Di-di-la scratched his ear and glanced to the side. Right hand up.

"Not really," he called back to Drom, with growing confidence. His tone alone brought a good number of eyes back to the battle.

A tiny shadow of doubt flickered across Drom's eyes, but he smiled widely and boomed,

"Well, I guess that we can't really define a reason at all then!"

Right hand up, twice. "Of course we can, s-s-silly!" cried out Di-di-la. This brought a titter from some of the monks sitting up close to the pavilion.

"Then is the definition..." huffed Drom, drawing himself up, "... not precisely..." he roared "...what I just said it was?" And he brought his hands down in a tremendous clap, right in front of Di-di-la's face.

Right hand, once, followed by my first two fingers, pointing apart. "Oh no, not at all," said Di-di-la, with a tasteful little touch of the tone you'd use to correct a child. The faces in the first ten rows were all glued on his now. "What you just gave is the definition of something else," continued Di-di-la. "Something t-t-totally different."

"And what would that be?" blustered Drom, stamping his foot with real anger now.

"Good," I said to myself. "Good. Nothing like a touch of anger to keep your mind from thinking straight." I held my hand out from under the shawl and joined the thumb and first finger in a circle, which in our country is like a thumbs-up.

"Why, what you gave was the definition of a *good* reason," replied Di-di-la, without a single stutter now. A good quarter of the monks had stopped their little conversations and were staring at him in disbelief. "A *reason*," Di-di-la concluded, on his own now, "is defined only as *anything which one gives as a reason*, whether it makes any sense or not.

"The mother of any young child could tell you that," he threw in, for good measure, and the crowd in the courtyard roared with delight. This was getting interesting.

Drom froze for the slightest moment, and his eyes fluttered up towards the three thrones, to the face of his uncle, the Founding Father. And I looked there too and saw a deadly glitter in the eyes; shouting wordlessly, "Crush him." Drom nodded slightly and turned back on Di-di-la like an enraged tiger—and the real battle began.

I can't tell you how long it went on, and I can't even tell you everything we said. The ideas flowed back and forth like bolts of lightning; clashing, thrusting, and counter-thrusting like blades in the hands of swordsmen. Centuries of wisdom flew by as we ripped apart the thoughts and insights and insights upon insights of generation after generation of the greatest sages of Mother India and her newborn child, Tibet.

And as much as I disliked so much of what he was, I can never deny that Drom rose fully to the challenge. He was brilliant, awesome, flying across the pavilion floor like nimble fingers on a loom, striking where he could and dodging when he had to, returning relentlessly. My hands flew back and forth like hummingbirds, and Di-di-la had to keep one palm up on his Geshe hat the whole time, covering the eyes fixed off to the side, on me.

Long-Life stared out his little peepholes, spellbound, a welcome warmth against my chest. Every once in a while I looked over Di-di-la's head at the occupants of the three thrones. The Precious One's face was aglow with pride for the warriors' performance. The Ancient One was looking on with obvious joy at the wonderful battle, his mouth wide open in a toothless grin. The Founding Father showed only a deadly and ever-growing concern that the contest was obviously so close; I could feel Drom feeling it, and the extra pressure every glance at the Founding Father put on the young man. And the Debate Master stood still and silent amidst it all, wrapped in his spectre's cloak.

Novices worked through the crowd and poured bowls of hot tea for monk and villager alike, but there was none for the warriors. By tradition they would go on, all night if they had to, without a moment's break—croaking out their questions and answers in parched voices as the battle wore on. Only one monk among all those assembled had the power to stop the warriors, and he was not the Abbot, the Founding Father, nor even the Ancient One. Only the Debate Master, only Geshe Lothar, could call the war to an end. And he would do so only when, in his mind, it was clear which warrior had prevailed; that is, unless one of the warriors gave him what we called The Look.

The Look was a very subtle thing, and a very sad thing. If a major battle were being fought in the courtyard—say a Geshe examination, or a contest between the champions of two different classes—a way out was always left open for the two warriors, in case one of them absolutely felt he could not go on. This saved the young men from a major embarrassment, and possibly a scar that might take a long time to heal, if they simply reached a point of exhaustion so unbearable that they could not continue. And it was all done in a split-second, so that oftentimes almost no one watching the battle even noticed it. You just caught the Debate Master's eye, in a certain way, and then let go immediately. A few minutes later he would call for the fight to end.

At some point the torches were lit—I didn't see it happen, I just realized that Di-di-la was straining to see my hands, and I looked around quickly and saw that it was all dark. There was a torch up on the gate post and I thrust my hands out from under the shawl into their light, as far as I could, without risking someone seeing me. At another point though I glanced around and saw that there was little danger of being spotted: there was not a single sound in the entire courtyard, nor among the crowd at the wall. Everyone was staring at the warriors, entranced by the flow of ancient words, even when they had no idea what they meant—and I can say that none of the villagers, and not that many even of the monks, could follow what was happening. It was more the rhythm of Drom's handclaps and the replies that Di-di-la threw back at them, and the dance of the attacker across the pavilion floor.

But the claps and the dance were wearing on Drom, and I saw it as the grueling hours passed. It was just the end of winter—the great debates were often scheduled to celebrate the welcome arrival of spring—and the night was turning frightfully cold. The monks looking on bundled up in their shawls and pulled their cloaks over their heads, and the villagers huddled closer, glad now for the warmth—but amazingly no one was even thinking of getting home. Drom though—Drom, never pausing, slashing and swinging long after his arms should have dropped from his body—was covered in sweat. Every hour or so in the middle of a question or a leap his hands would come up and rip another layer of ceremonial robes from his shoulders, cinching them around his waist like armor.

Blood was flowing freely over his hands from the powerful claps, and little droplets of red were splattered all over the front of Di-di-la's new golden robes. And then suddenly I noticed that the claps were getting fewer, and weaker, and I sensed that Di-di-la and I might be able to end the war, now, if we could hold on and strike even one really strong blow.

I took a good look at Di-di-la though and saw that it might already be too late. His head was drooping, and his voice was nearly gone. Somewhere during the last few exchanges, and I hadn't even noticed, he had dropped his hand completely from his hat and had his head turned directly towards me, looking for the answers and calling them out to Drom from the side of his mouth.

I held my palm up to my cheek and turned my head to the side, and Di-di-la caught it and switched his head back to Drom. But something was wrong there already; I saw Drom glance down at his friend Stick, and there was a quick exchange of the hand signals they'd been using for years at the courtyard to gang up on the other young men.

Stick nodded and looked up and started scanning the wall in my direction. I pulled my hands back as far as I possibly could. A few seconds later Stick nodded to Drom but then waved his hands to each side, as if to say there was nothing he could do, locked in on the far side of the crowd sitting up on the pavilion floor.

Then about a minute later there was a whole stream of signs from Stick and then from Drom to Hammer, who was squeezed into the last row on the near side. And then I saw Hammer's powerful form come up into a crouch, and one leg came down off the pavilion to the courtyard flagstones, and he dropped down into the first row there. He started picking his way through the rows, slowly, crouched like a cat, headed for the courtyard wall up towards the side of the pavilion. My heart stopped cold. If Di-di-la and I were going to pull this off, we had to do it in the next few minutes.

Drom had drawn himself up for a new attack, but he was obviously beginning to crack. The Founding Father's eyes—bright like embers— traced the young man's every move, critiqued his every word, darted this way and that in immediate judgment. And so when the final argument came, it was delivered in a voice that wavered with weariness and a growing fear of failing the Father.

35.

When One is Three

"Now all the things in our world, all the things around us," began Drom, "exist at one of three different layers, or levels." And he clapped his swollen hands one more time.

Left hand up at the wall: "That's correct," returned Di-di-la's tired voice.

"And things at the first layer are easy to perceive; things at the second layer are difficult to perceive; and those at the third layer are *very* difficult to perceive," droned Drom almost automatically, for this was a standard presentation from the old Indian textbooks on reasoning.

Left hand: "Again, correct," said Di-di-la, in a hoarse whisper.

After sending the sign I glanced off to my left—Hammer had nearly reached the wall, about fifty feet away from where I stood. "Hurry," I cried inside to Drom.

"And to perceive the things that are easy to perceive, we simply use our senses—our eyes, our ears, and so on. Or it could even be our minds when, for example, we listen to our own thoughts."

Drom had covered himself well; no sense making a stand at this point. Left hand up. "Correct," wheezed Di-di-la.

"And for things that are difficult to perceive, we must use reason—we must stop, and think, and figure them out, correct?"

Left hand. "Just so," nodded Di-di-la. I could judge Drom's fatigue just from the lack of controversy in the ideas he was laying out.

"And for things that are extremely difficult to perceive, well then we first find a person who we can establish is completely knowledgeable and truthful, and then ask them to tell us all of these things; am I right?"

Left hand. "Right." Hammer was having trouble getting down the wall through the crush of monks in the very back, but he was still no more than thirty feet away. I glanced around me desperately; there was nowhere to go, no way out. Behind me there was only the bulk of the giant farmer, and to each side a solid wall of monks. And I couldn't leave Di-di-la like that anyway. I turned to face the battle, for as long as I could.

"But isn't it true that it is quite impossible to give examples of the things that exist at each of the three layers?" asked Drom innocently, and I saw immediately where he was leading Di-di-la. But we had no choice but to go there, into a trap that might well mean our end, and not Drom's. And so right hand twice, cautiously. Hammer was held up only ten feet away, trying to step over a particularly stubborn clump of novices.

"No, not impossible at all," said Di-di-la, blissfully unaware of where that put us.

Drom raised one hand slowly, stiffly, and brought his hand down into a clap that sent a grimace of pain across his face. "*Sho!*" he cried, and spun around to show his back to Di-di-la. This was a warrior's way of saying that he didn't expect any good answer for quite some time. Coming around Drom held his head up to the wall, and spotted Hammer, and looked down the wall straight towards me, as if to say, "It's over."

Now the word *sho!* means what it sounds like—"Show me!"—which meant that Di-di-la would have to come up with good examples of the things at each of the three layers. This was no simple yes or no. The classical examples were in the ancient books: the color and shape of the sun was at the first level, easy to perceive. The fact that there is nothing in our whole life that has not come to us from how we have treated others is at the second level, difficult to perceive unless we can think it out carefully. And to perceive just what it was that we did long ago towards someone else which has now come back to us as any particular little detail of our life—a cold say, or even a cancer—this is extremely difficult, and we need the help of someone else, someone who knows. But all these were not something I could send on my hands to Di-di-la, and Drom knew it.

Hammer burst through; in a few strides he'd be on me. And then, under the pressure, my mind suddenly broke through to another level. I waved my hands in a big circle and mouthed "Everything."

Di-di-la looked back confused. Hammer was at my side, across the wall. I gave Di-di-la one last nod, calmly.

"Everything," he shouted back at Drom, sensing the impossibility of it all. "Everything. *Everything* is at *all three levels!*"

Drom turned around to face his enemy, with a look of utter disbelief.

"Everything?" he whispered.

"Everything," uttered Di-di-la, with finality.

Drom's face jerked in a strange spasm. "The words you just said," he croaked. "The words you just said. Are you telling me that even the words you just said exist at all three levels?"

Hammer's hand came up and tore the shawl from my head. I didn't even look at him. I raised my left hand, proudly, in the full light of the torch.

"That's right," said Di-di-la, and in that moment he grasped where we were going, and the rabbit led the lion to his downfall.

Drom didn't think; he just began taking Di-di-la through what we call the "check-back."

"Are you saying then that your words exist at the first level? Are you saying that what they mean is easy to perceive?"

Di-di-la nodded. "Yes," he said, and then he abruptly added: "And what you really should ask me now, my friend, is 'For whom?' Go ahead, ask it."

Drom stared at him in total exhaustion, entirely spent, and there was nothing else he could do.

"For whom?" he said.

"For me," said Di-di-la calmly, and pointed his finger to his own chest.

Drom continued dumbly down the checkback. "And do your words also exist at the second level—is their meaning, at the same time, also difficult to perceive?"

Di-di-la nodded again and mouthed "For whom?"

"For whom?" asked Drom, in strange obedience.

"For them, I think," said Di-di-la quietly, and gestured towards the wall, to the crowd of villagers.

I finally glanced at Hammer. He felt something coming. He was standing half turned to me and turned halfway back to the battle, his eyes fixed on Drom with a pained look, his hand on the wall, the other still in the air, clutching Grandmother's shawl.

"And do your words," breathed Drom, "do they simultaneously exist on the third level; is their meaning also something very difficult to perceive?"

Di-di-la nodded, without a word. His big scared eyes went to Drom's and drew the last words out.

"For whom?" said the warrior.

Di-di-la lowered his hand from his hat, slowly, ever so slowly, and he pointed. He pointed straight at Drom.

I saw the big boy's face change as he went through the choices. Agree that he didn't know what Di-di-la was talking about? Disagree, and say that he did, but had needed Di-di-la's help to do so, and so had asked his questions—and thus agree by disagreeing? And then something inside him broke, and one powerful shudder shook his whole body, and he just stood there, his strong shoulders heaving up and down, his eyes staring blankly at the ground.

"Well I... I mean... but..." and then he just stopped. The courtyard went into total silence, as silent as the cold glittering stars in the dark over our heads. A thousand faces fixed on the broad back and shoulders, pumping up and down, in jerks now, as if Drom were sobbing. But his eyes were dry, and I saw them, and they went up to the throne, the throne where the Founding Father sat bolt upright, his fist raised before his chest in frustration, and fury. And then the eyes dropped back to the ground, but somewhere on the way they paused, for the tiniest instant, and met Geshe Lothar's, and gave him The Look.

36.

The Sun Rises, from a Very Unexpected Place

The spectre, the Debate Master, stirred, for the first time in all those hours. The arm came straight out with the cloak, waving like the wing of some great eagle, and he called out. And his voice rang through the entire courtyard, and to the wall, and beyond it, far into the night, crying "*Oh... la... so!*" which is to say, "It is... ended!"

I brought my hands down to the cold stone of the wall, and only then realized they were completely numb with cold and the hours of holding them up to Di-di-la. Drom turned, and slumped down on the examination bench next to Di-di-la. He bent over and buried his face in his hands; thin little streams of blood started flowing down his arms from the cracks that had opened up between his fingers. Di-di-la sat up straight, just staring straight ahead, and instinctively brought his hand up and laid it on Drom's shoulder, to comfort him.

The Chanting Master, sitting in the first row up on the pavilion, began a few brief traditional prayers to conclude the battle. People started looking around to collect their things, and began to talk to their neighbors again. Monks around me were already beginning to ask each other why the Debate Master had stopped the contest in the middle of an argument. And I had already heard someone say "Maybe one of them gave him The Look?" when the chanting stopped, and Geshe Lothar did one of the kindest things I have ever seen anyone do.

It was years really before I fully realized how kind it was, for in a single moment he saved the Founding Father, and he saved Drom, and he saved Drom from the Founding Father, and he saved a lot of other people—saved us from years of hard feelings, recriminations, doubts, and pride—saved really the peace of our monastery. And it was all because he stepped, the spectre in the cloak; he stepped suddenly between the two young warriors, stood there between them, and silently placed a hand upon each one's shoulder. Then he turned and raised that stone face to the three thrones.

"A judgment!" exclaimed a young monk at my side. "The Debate Master has called... he's called for a judgment! He stopped it for a judgment!"

An excited murmur raced through the crowd, and those who had begun to stand sat down again suddenly, and the hands stopped moving and the voices fell silent. All eyes went up to the pavilion again, to the three thrones, and whatever rumors had begun died in their throats in that moment.

For the Debate Master had also this one further absolute power in the courtyard, in the courtyard where he had stood for thousands of hours, tirelessly, over the last ten years, bringing his young warriors into their strength. Only he could call for a judgment: only he could stop the battle, knowing that a Geshe had proven himself.

There was a terrible silent moment of suspense. Di-di-la's face was turned calmly up to the cold night sky, in sheer resignation. Drom's face never came out of his hands. And the spectre stepped again, directly behind Drom now, and put both his hands on those two powerful shoulders. The stone face turned again to the thrones.

The Precious One, the Abbot, had changed completely. His face was bathed in a soft golden light, a kind of absolute serenity and sacredness, like a very pure, young maiden. He turned his head slowly and looked over to the side, at the throng of villagers at the wall, and then in a kind of perfect grace carried his gaze across the entire courtyard and to the warriors seated on the timbers beyond. And then his back went straight as a rod, and his head came up in a look of pride for the wonder he had witnessed that night—a birth, really—and then he looked down into the stone eyes of the spectre and nobly nodded his head, once.

The spectre looked at the Founding Father, who nodded his head quickly, three or four times, in a quick nervous gesture. Then the Father's eyes, and the spectre's, and everyone else's fixed upon the Ancient One—for all three must agree.

The Ancient One's face burst out again into that huge toothless grin of joy, and he nodded happily, like a child asked whether he would like a piece of candy.

And still it was silent, totally silent. My heart began to pound, loudly, so loud I was sure everyone could hear it, and I felt I was going to faint. Long-Life stirred against my belly, gently, and it kept me there. The spectre moved to Di-di-la, and put his hands on the thin little shoulders. The boy dropped his head and stared nervously at the ground.

The Abbot smiled, and nodded. The Founding Father stared furiously at the faces of the other two, and then gave a curt nod. The Ancient One agreed to his candy, a second time. A Geshe had proven himself, as had another. The entire crowd, in a single voice, in a single instant, broke into a cheer of approval.

Just as suddenly a silence broke out, beginning from the pavilion and spreading to the last villager at the wall. The Ancient One was struggling up on his throne, trying to stand. But the hours of sitting and cold had left his legs useless — he waved his arms down at an attendant, who climbed the stairs to the throne and lifted the aged monk up to his feet bodily, and practically carried him down the stairs.

The Ancient One shuffled forward to the bench, and came around to the front, fumbling inside his robes for something. And then he pulled out a shining silken white *kata:* the long thin scarf of ceremonial greeting. He hobbled over to Drom and gently lifted the young man's face from his hands. There was a wide smudge of blood across one cheek, and he looked up at the Ancient One with glazed eyes.

The old monk patted him on the shoulder and reached up and softly wiped away the blood. And then he carefully draped the scarf around the big boy's neck, and hugged him, pressing his forehead against the top of Drom's head.

The crowd went wild. This was an ancient form of congratulations, and a high blessing, from the greatest warrior in our whole part of Tibet. The Ancient One held Drom for a long moment there like that, and then straightened up and looked him in the eye and gave him a proud nod. And that brought Drom out of it, and he looked up like a little boy, and with a wan smile thanked the old man.

Then the Ancient One stepped towards Di-di-la, but went on, to the side, without a word or a gesture. The little monk cast his eyes down, and I did too. And then I heard a murmur rising through the crowd, and looked up.

The Ancient One was standing at the side of the bench, on Di-di-la's side, looking harshly into the eyes of his attendant, who was still holding him up. The Ancient One was demanding something, and the attendant again refused. But then finally the old man just pulled his arm away and set both his hands down on the edge of the bench, and fell down on one knee there. And then he slowly took off his ancient Geshe hat and lowered his forehead, and touched it to the bench.

The crowd gasped as one. This was more than giving Di-di-la a blessing. It was *asking* for a blessing. The Ancient One was saying, without words, that Di-di-la had fought as well as any of the great warriors of the olden days, in Mother India. And when the head came back up the crowd broke into sheer pandemonium, a roar of excitement and happiness: happiness for the two young men, happiness for the monastery, happiness for the precious knowledge itself, and for all those who kept it alive in the world. Monks jumped up and rushed for the stage of the pavilion; others pulled off their Geshe hats and waved them wildly through the air as they danced in circles; villagers turned to hug each other in joy. I burst into tears of exhaustion, and relief, and elation, and sadness, wishing Tenzing were here, and Grandmother, to hug and dance with.

Long-Life felt the surge of the crowd and could simply no longer contain himself. He burst out of the baby sling and leaped onto the top of the wall, barking with joy to match the cheers of the people. He raced up and down the length of the wall, singing to the sky, with his long beautiful tail flying behind him—stopping at one point to leap up and snatch Grandmother's shawl out of Hammer's hand. Hammer stood staring at the little lion, and me, with a dull stunned look.

I couldn't help myself and just raised my head to the sky, laughing, and laughing, and crying and laughing—I couldn't stop. And maybe a few minutes or a few hours later I looked again to the pavilion. The Ancient One was being whisked away from the mob on the arms of three or four sturdy attendants. The Precious One was leaning back in his throne and regarding the whole melee with the look of an indulgent daddy. The Founding Father had come down the steps of his throne, and was standing with Drom off to the side. The young warrior's eyes were down, looking at the ground, and the Father was surveying him with a strange mixture of pride and disappointment.

Then I saw Stick come and stand between them. He took the Founding Father by the arm and put his mouth up to his ear and said some words, and then pointed over towards where I was standing. And then suddenly Stick was staring into my face with resentment; and Drom too was looking at me with a kind of angry pain; and I felt Hammer's eyes too like that, and finally the cold eyes of the Founding Father—waking into a realization of what had happened, slowly turned upon me, glowing in fury.

And then I did something that I know was not very wise—and it was another of those things that changes the course of our lives. I raised my head proudly, in the torchlight, so that the eyes, all those eyes, would know who I was, and never forget. And then I grabbed Long-Life in my hands, and whispered in his ear "Sorry little lion; just this once." And I turned him around then on the top of the wall, and grabbed hold of his tail, and lifted it up, to show the Father and the terrible trio exactly where the sun had just come up from.

And then I took one last long sweet look at my dear brother Di-di-la, still sitting there on the bench, surrounded by a mob of delighted monks pounding him on the shoulders. Then I whirled away from the wall, and there was the face of the giant farmer—very red now—and he opened his mouth to say something, but my baby and I were already gone, dancing through the crowd to the horse road.

37.

I See Myself, Halfway

We walked briskly down the horse road;
Uncle I knew would be tied up with people
congratulating him for his fine work with the two
warriors, but it was still better to be home and back
in my sickbed long before he returned. I got Long-
Life back in the sling but let him sit with his paws
on the front to get the night air—the masquerade
was over. I pulled Grandmother's scarf down
around my shoulders against the cold, and only
then did it slowly dawn on me what had just
happened. All the years of work—all the silent
singing with Tenzing; all the little notes at the
window; the endless debates with cows and dogs
and looms; the years at the courtyard wall, ever
since that first trip with Grandmother—it was all
over.

And I had done what everybody said that girls just don't do: I had learned the Five Great Books, I knew the Wheel of Life; and even if no one—or nearly no one—ever found out, I had stood in the final battle, and earned the golden hat of a Geshe: a hat which, I reflected wryly, would never touch my head.   And with these thoughts of contentment, over an impossible job well done, I walked, in the cold—happy at times to hear the excited voices of the villagers around me, as they recounted to each other the feats of the warriors.

But before we reached the tree, to recover the little rug, my thoughts had begun to darken. Something was on my mind, something was tugging at it, holding it back from the golden stream of happiness and accomplishment. Faces came to me, one by one—the faces at the very end. Stick, and then Drom, and then Hammer and the fury of the Founding Father. But I realized that this wasn't where my mind was stuck. And it took me all that long walk to face what was really wrong.

It was Di-di-la. It was Di-di-la's face—the look on his face, there at the very end, sitting on the bench in the midst of a mass of golden robes and cheers and handshakes. I looked again at my memory of his face—I forced myself to look—and then I knew. For it was not a face of happiness, nor any face of joyful achievement. It was a face of

379

anguish, the special pain of the guilty, of people who have a secret, a bad secret.

And then I just stopped there, in the middle of the road, and people flowed around me and looked back at me, and Long-Life turned with sad eyes and looked up too, knowing something was wrong; but I didn't see any of them. I just saw Di-di-la's face, and in an instant of pain and remorse it came to me: I had taken away his Geshe hat—I had denied him his hat—and not to help him really; maybe not to help anyone, really: just to prove that I could do it, just to do what people had told me I couldn't do. And I stood there in the road seeing too much of myself in the dark and tiredness; and I started to weep, and wept all the way home, and wept myself to sleep.

I woke in the morning late, with the dull headache that people get when they haven't slept enough. My forehead was hot, and my nose was running, and I guessed I was coming down with a cold—maybe from the hours at the wall the night before; maybe from the doubts that had filled me since. I hurried to dress and go make the tea, but then remembered what Uncle had said, about the meeting with the visitors, and knew he wouldn't be back for hours.

I did take Amala her very late tea, but she didn't seem to mind. She was in unusually good spirits—still not talking, but sitting up straight on her cushion at the loom, toying with the colored threads of the same old carpet. At first I thought that the visit from the caravan women the night before must have cheered her up, but then I thought that maybe she had sensed something of the wonderful battle. And that took my thoughts to Tenzing, and that took them to Di-di-la, and that led me into a gloom that was not so wonderful, and I sat there with Amala for a long time, watching her smile at the colors of the yarn, bright now in a shaft of golden light from the sky-window. And then I knew what I had to do.

The day seemed to stand still as I waited for Uncle to come home. I was going to tell him everything, everything I had done to prove them all wrong. And I was going to admit that it wasn't all for the healing; not for Grandmother, not for Tenzing even, or Amala—because I knew now, I really knew, that a lot of it had just been selfish. And it had caused my new brother Di-di-la to lose what little self-esteem he had ever had.

I made Uncle a nice lunch, but noon came and passed and there was still no sign of him; finally I just shared it among the yaks and cows—I was too nervous to eat, one moment sure that I could bare my soul to Uncle, another moment deciding that a partial confession would probably be enough, with different parts left out as the hours wore on. It was nearly dark, and I was out at the loom weaving nothing, starting to sniffle and sneeze in the gathering cold, before I heard his steps.

All my resolve vanished in that single moment. I greeted Uncle as cheerfully as I could, and he stood at the door to his yurt looking very tired and inquired about my health, and I said I was almost completely better, and he nodded and went inside. I brewed him a strong tea with lots of nutmeg to make him happy, and then I went in with the churn. I poured out a cup for him and set it on the table, and took one look at that weary, noble face, and I broke into tears and sat down there on the rug halfway up on my knees, and everything poured out of me, everything I'd ever done, beginning from the songs with Tenzing and ending with the insult to the Founding Father and his warriors.

Uncle listened in silence, staring at his silent hands rested on his lap. The tea went cold, and the sun went down, and the only light was the soft golden glow of the butter lamps on the altar. And when it was done I stayed there still, feeling the cold sweeping through my knees, weeping and sniffling. Uncle was quiet for a long time, and then he stirred himself.

"But Friday, why are you so sad? You stretched the rules, you pushed the boundaries, but after all you have accomplished something very extraordinary, and all to learn the healing—all to help others, to help people like Grandmother, and Tenzing, and Amala. Why are you so sad?"

I looked up and it came into my mind to tell Uncle how much I really knew—how much I really knew about myself, how much I knew about why I had done everything, how much of it was just my pride, just my stubbornness, just my selfishness really. But that part was so hard, so hard to tell, and it wouldn't come out at all. In the end I couldn't admit it even to myself, much less to Uncle. And so I did half a confession, as I had done half a Geshe.

"It's... it's Di-di-la, Uncle. After it was all finished, while I was walking home, I realized... I realized that he will have to live, live like that, his whole life—never knowing, never knowing if he could have done it by himself, never knowing if he had really earned the name, the name of 'Geshe' that people will call him for the rest of his life."

Uncle nodded slowly, and looked me straight in the eyes, willing the rest to come out. But it was stuck there, stuck there by my pride, and I just lowered my eyes to the floor in silence. And then it was quiet, for a long time, and Uncle finally sighed and took a sip of the cold tea, and cleared his throat.

"And so," he whispered thoughtfully, gazing straight ahead, "and so... things are not what they seem."

Then he looked me in the face again, and said, "Some things have happened... some things have happened at the monastery—some things you should know.

"Right after the battle last night, Di-di-la went straight to the Debate Master's quarters and confessed that he had not earned his Geshe hat— that someone in the crowd had been helping him the whole time, with secret hand signals. He gave the hat back to the Debate Master. Then in the morning he went to the Precious One, the Abbot, and confessed to him. And today, after the meetings of the visiting Lamas and the Council of Elders, he repeated his confession to me, to his teacher," Uncle sighed heavily.

I sat stunned, knowing how much pain I had caused. I started to cry again.

Uncle reached down and patted me on the shoulder. "Wait, he said with a bit of gloomy cheer, "that's not the end of it.

"The Precious One took me aside afterwards and we had a long talk. We were both aware that the Founding Father was extremely agitated all through the meetings this morning, and that he seemed especially upset at me, for some reason. So we surmised that he must have caught wind of something about a person helping Di-di-la, but strangely he wasn't saying a peep about it. And Di-di-la steadfastly refused to name his accomplice, saying that it was all his own idea, and his own fault, and that he didn't feel he had the right to confess for anyone else.

"But then Geshe Lothar came in and spoke at length with the Precious One; and the Precious One himself—you know—he doesn't let on, but he's an extremely perceptive man. You have to be," sighed Uncle again, "to run a monastery that has so many younger monks."

Uncle took another sip of his cold tea and made a face; I poured him a fresh one. "And after all this the Precious One decided, first of all, that there was no sense making a big fuss about it all—particularly with the visitors here—and especially if the Founding Father himself preferred to keep the whole thing quiet. It seems that, er... well... frankly, the Father would rather have people believe that Di-di-la whipped his nephew, than for everyone to find out that it was really just a certain young country girl." He smiled down at me, for the first time, and I was ever so grateful.

Then Uncle cleared his throat again and went on a little more smoothly, as if he were conducting a class and leading his young charges through an extended line of reasoning.

"Now that still left this problem of a Geshe who wasn't really a Geshe running around the monastery for the rest of his life, and so the Precious One and Geshe Lothar took Di-di-la into an empty room up on top of the temple and grilled him for a good three hours on the Five Great Books, and the Wheel of Life. He came out looking like a bag of barley squeezed through a millstone, but from all accounts he did splendidly, and the Abbot has delivered a private judgment that Di-di-la is truly Geshe material. And so they made him take the hat back, and issued him his punishment, and sent him home to get some rest."

"Issued... a punishment?" I said sadly.

"Oh yes," said Uncle firmly. "No way they could let someone get away with cheating like that! Di-di-la has pulled what I guess has to be the longest kitchen duty ever awarded to a newly capped Geshe. Three years of helping to cook, and washing *all* the dishes!" Uncle gave a hearty laugh.

"All?" I whispered unbelievingly. "All the dishes? For hundreds of monks? For three whole years?" I gazed down at the floor. "But that means... that means he will never be able to come out here to the homestead, to help you... to learn more from you." And that seemed like the hardest punishment of all.

"On the contrary!" boomed Uncle, like a junior Geshe Lothar. "Di-di-la's kitchen duty is to be performed here, at our kitchen, here at the homestead!"

My jaw dropped in astonishment. And then my mind turned around and ran the other way and I said, "But Uncle—we don't have more than about ten dishes here anyway."

"Not *yet,*" Uncle corrected me, "but we will have, once the School gets started!" He beamed and waited for me to blurt back,

"What school, Uncle?"

"Our new school for the villagers—the school where we teach them the steps!"

"What steps, Uncle?"

"The Steps of the Way!" he rushed back. "An idea I've been working on for years—a summary of the Five Great Books, but for people who don't have time to be a monk; for people who are busy with their lives and families but who really want to know about what the monks learn, about the Wheel of Life and everything! And so we'll have a little school, here at the homestead, and any villager—man or woman alike—who wants to come can come and learn, in their spare time, in the evening; and they'll all get this nice class and a cup of tea and a little snack, everything free, everything happy!"

"Where are you going to do all this, Uncle?" I exclaimed.

"Oh! Just so! No problem! Before your father left on this last trip he promised me a big new yurt, for Di-di-la to sleep in, and as a place to hold the classes, and all the kitchen things, if I could succeed in getting this idea past the Council of Elders, and the Founding Father! And by golly, just this morning, everything got approved! And through a real miracle the Awakened Ones have even sent our kitchen help!"

I thought for a moment, and then said suspiciously, "I can't believe you got all this past the Founding Father, Uncle, especially if he was in such a terrible mood this morning."

Uncle looked a little sheepish. "Well, when he heard that both I and Di-di-la would be doing all the teaching…"

I raised my eyebrows.

"He's a Geshe, my dear Friday! And that's what new Geshes do—they start helping with the teaching. And there's no way I can cover my regular classes *and* the School, *and* the Project…"

"*Project?*" I burst in.

"Later dear, one thing at a time," he smiled, looking into the future with joy. "So when the Founding Father heard that Di-di-la and I would be stuck out here—closer to the village, so more people can come—he immediately realized that this would keep both of us out of his hair at the monastery practically forever. And so he looked like he might go along with the idea… but, to tell you the truth…" Uncle stumbled a bit, which raised my suspicions even further.

"The truth?" I repeated, waiting for it.

"Well… to tell you the truth… what really swayed the Founding Father, and the whole Council really, was the Ancient One. He'd been invited to sit in on our meeting, and when he heard about the idea of the school for villagers," here

Uncle began pouring out everything real fast, like an excited little kid, "well he just burst out and said it was the greatest idea he'd ever heard of and said he was going to start one up too over near his monastery and would need copies of the little book I've prepared and..." Uncle was radiant with the memory. "And well, frankly, the Founding Father didn't really have any choice," he said flatly, "no choice at all."

"Amazing," I breathed.

"What's that?" asked Uncle.

"Amazing," I said again, "that the only Lama who can outweigh even the Founding Father shows up on the same day that the Council discusses your new idea, Uncle! Why, I don't believe the Ancient One has even been in this whole area for years!"

Uncle reddened perceptibly. "Oh, yes, yes, amazing. A true stroke of fortune," he paused, and then looked up brightly. "And so everyone went along, even the Founding Father!" I gazed up with a look of love and amusement. So we were birds of a feather, after all.

Then Uncle's face went very serious, and he frowned, and he said very gravely, "But that man— the Founding Father. He's mad as a hornet, and he can be very dangerous when he's angry, you know. And so you and I are going to have to tread lightly for quite some time—agreed?"

I nodded. I understood just how serious it could be, and how many wonderful things were at stake now.

"The issue about that last battle, and Drom, and all that," began Uncle, "now that's not such a big deal. Thanks to Geshe Lothar, almost no one but the Founding Father realizes how badly Drom was defeated, and that he had to resort to The Look.

"And Drom and Di-di-la will still meet again, next week—after all the other candidates have had their battles. That will be to decide whether either of them deserves an *angi:* to be a Geshe of highest rank, or even second or third rank, of distinction.

"And to be very honest with you, Drom will destroy Di-di-la when Di-di-la plays the attacker: there's no way anyone can help him. We just have to hope," said Uncle with a trace of worry, "we just have to hope that Di-di-la doesn't do so poorly that people begin to demand that he be stripped of his new hat." Uncle paused again, mentally calculating the odds of a total disaster.

"And so the whole world will see what the Founding Father wants them to see—that his pride and joy is the greatest of the new Geshes. And Drom really is very good, and we all know that he deserves at least one of the ranks—probably third, or even second, I'd guess. And the Founding Father knows all this, and it will happen like that, and things will settle down.

"But I want you to give me your promise, my little bag of trouble, that you will steer clear of Drom and the Father, and not give them even the slightest excuse to cause any problems. It's your family at stake, Friday, their very safety; and more than that now, with the School. You realize that."

I nodded, and I really meant it, and Uncle saw it. He nodded too.

"And so you and me, this whole next week, we're going to sit quiet here at the homestead, and not even get close to the courtyard until all the battles among Tenzing's classmates are done and over with. Do I make myself clear?"

I nodded again, a little slower. Miss out on Di-di-la's last debate?

"Of course, at the end of the week, we will still have to go and see that last debate, the one between Drom and Di-di-la," said Uncle, with a touch of defiance.

I raised my eyebrows again.

"Well, we have to go, don't we? Why, he's family! Not even the Founding Father can deny us that!" exclaimed Uncle.

And I got up and gave my dear old uncle a huge hug of joy, and collected the churn and the cup, and went to the door.

"Er... Friday... just a minute," said Uncle then.

38.

Hats and Rugs

"Come," he said gently, "come and sit down again."

I came, and Uncle fumbled around in his things for a moment. Then he pulled out a worn saffron-colored cloth, and set it in his lap, and opened it with loving care. Inside was his Geshe hat, the lovely old one from Mother India.

He took the hat and held it in his hands for a long moment, as though saying farewell to an old friend. And then he reached out and placed it in my own hands.

"Congratulations," he said simply. "You have done me proud; you have done the family proud—and... and I'm sure Grandmother and Tenzing would have been especially proud."

I blushed deeply, but smiled deeply too, as we do at such moments—and then I held the hat back to him. "Oh no Uncle, no, really, I can't. Your beautiful hat... ."

"Oh no problem," he said cheerfully, "I can get another one from the monastery. They've got tons of them."

"No Uncle, really, I can't..." I stood up and tried to push the hat back into his hands.

"No, take it," he insisted. "You've earned it—earned it with the half."

I blushed again. "Oh Uncle, it wasn't all me; I... I couldn't have done it without you... without the classes."

Uncle surveyed my face sternly. "That's not the half that I was talking about. I mean what you did today, not last night. This is the stuff that Geshes are made of; this is what we try to learn."

And he waited again for the other half, but my pride kept me now even from seeing my pride, and the hat in my hands somehow made it worse. I glanced to the floor.

"It will come," said Uncle quietly. Then he laughed and said, "But you have to promise me, Geshe Friday, that the only person who ever sees you with that hat on is Long-Life!"

I laughed then too, and it was enough for one day, and I wrapped the hat in the cloth with reverence, and went to take my rest.

In the morning I took Uncle his tea; he looked bright and chipper, completely refreshed. When I set the churn down he glanced up from a big piece of parchment on his lap and burst out, "Niece... I mean *Geshe* Friday! I think all that debating has addled your brains!"

I smiled and poured out the tea. "Why so, Uncle dear?" The tension had left me too, and I felt light, full of sunshine.

"Why, I mentioned a special project yesterday, and you've forgotten to snoop around and figure out what it is!"

In truth I hadn't forgotten; and actually, I just hadn't gotten around to the snooping part yet. After all, it was only a bit past dawn.

"So what is this special project, Uncle?" I decided to try the direct approach for once.

He laughed and motioned for me to sit on the floor at the side of his bed. Then he took the parchment and turned it around and held it up for me to see.

"We... that is, I and all the translators I've trained... we are going to undertake an extraordinary project! We are going to translate the rest of the sacred books from India into our own language, and arrange them logically into a standard collection of knowledge that can be used by others for generations to come!"

"But Uncle," I said, "You've never taught anyone the Mother Tongue."

"Not so far!" he beamed. "But that's all going to change now. Yesterday the council also approved a school for translators, with the first classes to be held..."

"Here at the homestead," I finished for him, "in the morning, in your yurt, while Di-di-la teaches the beginner classes of the Geshe courses in his new yurt."

Uncle looked genuinely confused. "How... how did you know? Who told you? Come to think of it, I haven't told anyone else about all that yet myself!" Then he stopped and smiled. It was hard to be as much of a do-gooder as Uncle, but not so hard to guess where his do-gooding would lead to next. I looked more closely at the parchment he was holding up.

It was divided into red squares in a beautiful red ink we have that comes from a plant called *sel*. Each square was divided again with a diagonal line, also in red. On each side of this line was written a letter—something in Sanskrit, the Mother Tongue, on the upper left; and then down on the right a letter in our own language, Tibetan. I guessed what it was and nodded in appreciation, and Uncle nodded back, grateful for the appreciation.

"Right," he said. "Same sounds in each box. Great for teaching my new translators the alphabet of the Mother Tongue. Problem is, I can't get a parchment big enough for the whole thing. I want to put it on the wall, you see—" he jumped up and held it on the wall over near the altar "—so that people sitting in the class can just glance up and see the letter they need there, all big and clear, without having to get up themselves, or squint."

"And so I figured..." he said suggestively, but this time I couldn't see where he was headed.

"Well," he went on, excitedly, "I figured, well, you know, with the whole week off now, and no classes the whole time, I figured that you and me—well, more *you* really—I figured, well, Friday, would you be willing to weave all this into a big beautiful rug, for me, for the Project?"

My heart leaped. There was nothing that would please me more, especially since I knew that the ancient books of the thread sages—the keys to the other half of the healing—were all written in the Mother Tongue. And then slowly it dawned on me that the King was keeping his promise—his promise to teach me the sage's way, if I could finish even half of a Geshe's exam. And he was keeping his promise even without breaking his old promise *not* to teach me, because this business with the Mother Tongue all had the blessing of the Council and even the Founding Father—and certainly not even the Founding Father could expect Uncle to weave this rug on his own. My eyes got all wet again.

"Oh Uncle, yes, yes, of course, yes!" And I jumped up and hugged him.

We started right after lunch. Uncle came outside to my loom at the window—my invisible classroom for all those years—and sat with me, going through my box of yarns and picking out all the colors for the lines, the letters, and the background. His lap was covered with spools and then suddenly he said "Oops!" and looked up at me.

"What's wrong, Uncle?"

"Forgot the parchment!" he laughed, holding out his hands helplessly at the piles of yarn.

"Oh I'll fetch it for you, Uncle," I said, getting up.

"Up on the altar," he called, as I stepped to his door.

I walked over to the altar and took the parchment in my hands. There was a loose leaf of an old manuscript laying on the altar beneath it, which was odd. It was very unlike Uncle to leave any pages lying around: our books have no bindings, you see, and if you're not careful to wrap your pages back up in their wrapping cloth as soon as you're done reading, they tend to get lost and you end up with only half a book. Out of curiosity, I bent down to read the page—something any Geshe would have done, after all.

"The time for practice," it said, "once a person is already trained sufficiently, is when the third watch of the night has progressed some way; that is, so that the day breaks during the session." I looked up then, wrapped in thought. We Tibetans, a thousand years ago, we didn't have clocks and all that—although there was a kind of special cup which dropped water at a certain speed and ran out in an hour. But nobody used it—we divided one whole day and night into six periods, or watches, and we always knew where we were in each watch, just by glancing at the sun, or at the moon or the stars. We were also pretty good at just waking up in whichever part of a watch we'd decided to when we went to bed. Maybe Uncle was trying to tell me something, without telling me.

"Can't find it? he called again, from my side of the window. "Right there on top of the altar; can't miss it!"

I smiled and called back "Got it," and ran to begin the Mother Tongue.

I knew I'd have to work hard to finish the carpet within a week, but I also knew that weaving the shapes of the new letters would force me to learn them perfectly, the same way I'd done with Amala's designs. And so it went, with Uncle out by the loom every few hours, telling me that I had to tear out this or that section, and do it over, to get a letter just right—until they were all burned into my brain, indelibly. This is the way the Lamas work.

39.

Elder Sage

Long-Life and I woke up that night long before the third watch even began. I kept checking the stars and walked once or twice in the freezing cold over towards the family yurt, to see if there was any light leaking out of Uncle's window. And then just when I'd about given up hope, and was ready to crawl back under the warm covers, it came—a thin little sheet of gold, burning like a very warm welcome. We bundled up and padded soft as leopards over to Uncle's, around the back to the window, crouching there the same way we had when the young sage had gotten the instructions for his journey. It seemed like years ago, and not just months.

I raised my eyes to the shelf—the window flap had been pulled a bit to the side, and the room was bright with the light of a little row of butter lamps on the altar. Uncle was standing by the bed, with his back to me, in the yellow skirt and sleeveless top that the monks wear under their robes. He was tying something up under the skirt, at his waist. And then he reached, and pulled his shirt off; I had never seen him like that, without his usual layers of robes, and I wondered at the sleek strong look of his back, like Tenzing's, like the back of a youth of sixteen years. And then the skirt dropped, and he turned around, dressed now only in the simple, pure white loincloth of a thread sage. He looked the same in the front, young and strong, and his face was graced with a serene look of contemplation, pure concentration.

He bent over his bed, picked up a long white loop of cord there, and placed it with infinite grace over one shoulder, and around the other waist. I shivered to think how cold he had to be. He turned silently and sat down on the floor next to the altar—perhaps his eyes flickered towards the window, but perhaps not. I realized that he felt that he should never know for sure whether or not he was teaching me.

There silently in the middle of a long, thin cotton mat Uncle prayed for quite some time, sitting very still, his back as straight as an arrow. Then he sang some holy words, and afterwards cleared his nose in a way I'd never seen before, taking quick breaths and pushing the air out his nostrils in little explosions, sometimes blocking one side of his nose by pressing it with a finger, then switching and pressing the other side.

Then he stood up quickly and lightly, like a cat, and touched his forehead to the altar, and stood there in reverence. From there he stepped to the front edge of the cotton mat and stood very still, and quiet, and very straight, the way he'd been during his meditation. He looked straight ahead and seemed to be collecting his thoughts; then his breathing began to change, flowing in and out smoothly with a sort of rustle from deep within his throat. And then he began to dance.

I don't mean to say that it was the kind of dance that Grandmother Tara would have done at one of Father's bonfires. This was different, completely different—completely silent, flowing, graceful. Uncle's face would turn in a certain direction and then his eyes would come up and lock into a splendid gaze of concentration and his arms would move in a certain way, or he would crouch or stretch his legs, and then freeze there with the same smooth hoarse sound of his breath coming and going, peaceful but strong. And then according to some rhythm he would spring or slide slightly into another movement, freezing again into his breathing, until the rhythm demanded that he move again.

And even though I had no idea what he was doing, or what it was supposed to do for him, and for the healing, I could sense a sort of effect coming over him, circling around upon itself: his arms and his legs and other parts of his body would move in a certain way, and then following after the movements you could almost see a ripple or wave of energy move through him. And this energy seemed all to flow ahead into his mind, deepening his already very deep focus; and then in turn the focus, his concentration, would direct the body to move again, completing the ever-deepening cycle. And I was entranced by the cycles, and I have no idea how much time went by before suddenly Uncle had stopped, and gone briefly back into some silent prayers, sitting now as he had at the very beginning.

And then finally he stood, and went to his bed, and laid there quietly; but I could still feel the focus and energy coming from him, and I knew that this too must be some part of his practice. Then lastly he rose again, and put on his underskirt and shirt, and turning from the window again reached underneath and removed the white loincloth and then the thread. And then he blew out the lamps, and the yurt was dark, but over its top I could see the light of dawn just beginning to break.

Long-Life and I walked stiff and quiet back to our yurt, and I sat down near the fire pit there to think over what I'd seen. Except for the prayers—the focus, and the concentration—what I'd watched Uncle do was like nothing I'd ever heard of in all the classes he had taught me through the window. If I thought about it, it was almost like he was using his body to shape his mind a certain way, the patterns he weaved with his arms and legs and the rest almost suggesting patterns of thought to the mind within. And knowing Uncle's extraordinary depth in the many different ancient books and ideas, I had to believe that his mind too was weaving counter-thoughts to mesh and meld with those suggested by his body, and so from the outside and from the inside forces were set in motion to create a third thing—some very beautiful and holy thing, but I didn't know enough even to guess what it might be; only that it must have something very important to do with the healing: with stopping sickness, and the process of aging, and the Lord of Death himself.

But how was I to learn? I guessed that Uncle at this point just wanted me to watch, and perhaps imitate as well as I could what I could see with my eyes, and then—knowing Uncle—there was a plan of where things would go from there. And so with a few hearty yawns and the excitement of embarking on something big and new and important—that lovely but innocent excitement, so blissfully ignorant of the months and years of hard work ahead—I went back to my bed, already warmed by a tired, softly snoring little lion.

40.

I Get Dis-Invited

It was perhaps the most wonderful week of my entire life. Well before dawn I would rise and go with my erstwhile companion to watch Uncle, who never again even glanced towards the window. Each day I tried to pay special attention to one small part of his incredible dance, and then when I got back to my yurt I practiced it over and over again. Long-Life was a real gentleman and stayed awake to keep me company as I stumbled through something like the movements that Uncle's body sang so elegantly. I had no idea of how I was supposed to do the breathing exercises, and so I just did some loud, enthusiastic snorting that raised Long-Life's eyebrows.

As for the prayers, the meditation, I again had no way to know what Uncle was seeing, who he was talking to. But it seemed very natural just to go on praying to Gentle Voice, the Angel of Wisdom, asking help for the young monk whose name had come from the Angel's prayer itself: *di-di-di*. I had the seed of an idea about something that I could do for the big day—no helping with the hand signs or anything like that, of course—and I kept Tenzing's beautiful beads up on the altar near the little clay figurine of the Angel. Just about every day I placed a fresh little batch of dried cheese up there too, in Grandmother's little red pouch.

About halfway through the week, and most of the way through Uncle's special rug, some of the men from the caravan camp came riding in, leading several yaks loaded with poles and big sheets of felt. Uncle stepped out to greet them, and led them over to a specific spot across from his yurt. Uncle did some prayers over the ground, pouring sacred water from a small beautiful bronze pitcher. And then by evening his new schoolhouse, and Di-di-la's home and extra kitchen, were standing proudly at the edge of the clearing, our four yurts forming a square now.

Uncle called me over to the new yurt then; I got up slowly from my weaving and ambled across. I was a bit sore from practicing Uncle's dance—I am not inclined at all to physical exercise, being more interested in books and such, and never would have dreamed of trying to follow the dance, except that I sensed deep in my heart that it was very important for learning to heal myself and others. It was also making a mess of all my long *chuba* dresses, as I had to roll them or fold them or even tie them up in all sorts of odd places as I went through Uncle's movements. I was dying to get a close look at that white loincloth so I could try making one for myself, but I had no idea where Uncle kept it, and he practically never left his yurt anyway.

Uncle took me on a little tour of the spacious new yurt: the fire pit, the pots and pans, and Di-di-la's simple furniture. Then he sat me down and said, "There are some things coming up after the last battle at the courtyard that you should know about; I'm going to need your... ah... cooperation. It's very important." I nodded and Uncle went on.

"Now Di-di-la's last debate will be held three days from now, on the eighth day of the growing moon."

I nodded again. This was considered a very lucky day, what with the new light in the night sky halfway to its fullness.

"The day after that is a day of celebration; it's a tradition for everyone to go to visit with the new Geshe, and sit and have a cup of tea, and enjoy their accomplishment with them. I thought you and I could go to Di-di-la's together," Uncle smiled, and I smiled back warmly. It sounded like a lot of fun, and I was curious to see what Di-di-la's room at the monastery looked like.

"Now as for visiting Drom," continued Uncle, and from the seriousness in his voice I knew that this was the real reason why we were talking, "we're going to do something different. You know that I... that I had a certain responsibility to train Drom especially, and that your father... he... well, generously committed to helping Drom hold a rather... well, rather substantial ceremony with all the monks, to celebrate the successful conclusion of his studies. You know too that your father will then be making a significant contribution, through the Founding Father, to help construct a new main temple at the monastery.

"And so your father and I, to plan all this, and to sort of patch things up with the Founding Father—which I dare say is even more important now after that *last* battle in the courtyard—" here Uncle's eyes twinkled a bit, "we've arranged for Drom and his uncle to come out to the homestead on the next day after that, to have a nice long dinner and spend a comfortable night here, and then discuss all the arrangements for the contributions, on the following morning."

I raised my eyebrows in surprise; Uncle looked a little uncomfortable, but forged ahead.

"Now your father has sent word that his caravan is close enough to home now that he is sure he'll be in early that very morning for the discussions; this means that all you and I have to worry about is the dinner, and making sure the Founding Father and his new Geshe get a peaceful sleep the night before."

Here Uncle paused and glanced nervously down at his tea cup, signaling that he was about to get to the real meat of the matter. Then suddenly it dawned on me what he was about to say.

"Uncle dear," I said with a wry smile, "I believe you are about to tell me that—at least until my golden-tongued father has appeared—I should be sure not to show my face outside my yurt the whole time the Founding Father is within, say, two or three miles of the homestead; am I right?"

Uncle nodded gratefully.

"No problem," I said, feeling a little defensive. "I want to see them about as much as they want to see me. But what are you going to do about the meals? I can't see Amala cooking all that, especially not here in Di-di-la's yurt, in front of the Founding Father."

Uncle nodded and went down one of his logic paths. "Got that covered already. I talked to the men today and confirmed it. You remember our old milkmaid—Bukla—well she's got a sister named Mutik who it seems is a wonderful cook and an excellent conversationalist, which might make up for... well, for me. And so she's agreed to come over and be our dinner cook and hostess."

I glanced down at the ground; Uncle gave a little laugh. "Come come now, my dear Geshe. You can't run a man through with your sword and then expect him to appreciate it when you throw him a dinner party. The best thing you can do for all of us is to lay low. Agreed?"

I nodded, and then Uncle did an old warrior's trick of changing the subject right away. "Now we're just about done with the weaving of the Mother Language, right?" he asked.

I went gracefully with him. "Yes, Uncle; and a few days early!" Then I saw his eyes brighten up, and knew I shouldn't have said that. In the past several days he had already added a good three feet of "very useful other stuff."

"Excellent! Well then we have time to throw in the combination letters!" And he dragged me to his yurt and produced another sizable parchment that he "just happened to have ready." It contained an addition to the first chart with all the very odd combination letters that are often formed when two single letters of the Mother Tongue bump into each other.

I nodded with a helpless smile, and admiration, and gave Uncle a look that said, "Is that really all there's going to be?"

"Oh yes," he replied. "That's it. That's absolutely it. All you need to be able to read anything at all in the Mother Language…" and then he gave me a strange, thoughtful look "… although of course you wouldn't know what it meant, until you'd been trained by a real Master."

And he gazed off in the direction of the window, and the die was cast.

41.

Inside

On the big day Uncle and I left some of the caravan women with Amala and then started off along the short-cut over the slate ridge: the route that Uncle always took to the monastery when he was in a hurry. Not that we were late, but Uncle was all nerves again and wanted to be extra sure that he got a good seat in the row reserved for the senior teachers. I had chosen to wear a simple old dress of mine, partly in protest of the finery that most people would, and partly to help reinforce my new image as a quiet and obedient country girl.

I wore Tenzing's beads around my neck, as any other country girl would wear theirs, and the turquoise mother bead tapped against my nervous heart as we walked along. The stone felt warm there, almost hot, as if it were charged with some

kind of wonderful power from all the prayers I'd
done over it. Long-Life walked alongside me until
we were past the ridge, and then let me know that
he expected to be carried the rest of the way in the
baby sling. My little lion was becoming a real
aristocrat's lapdog, but I enjoyed pampering him—
as did the whole family, especially when he did his
tricks at mealtimes.

The wall around the courtyard was already
nearly filled with villagers as we arrived; Uncle left
me at a pretty good spot not far from the gate,
which put me almost directly behind the attacker's
back. Then as he turned to enter the courtyard,
Uncle threw one last significant glance towards my
hands, for added emphasis, and I nodded back
with my new obedient-style smile.

If the crowd before had been large, this one
was massive, by the time the great gong was
sounded. Drom and Di-di-la's was the final battle
of the Geshe examinations for the year, since the
first pair to fight did their second debate last—and
no one had forgotten their opening encounter.
Four other warriors had been awarded Geshe hats,
including both Stick and Hammer. Stick had done
so well during his second battle that the judges had
granted him the extra distinction of third rank, and
our class leader—the quiet sincere one—had
earned a second rank. Two such awards were
considered exceptional for one year's new crop of

Geshes, and Drom would really have to work today if he hoped to win any extra rank at all. As for Di-di-la, we were all just hoping for a graceful defeat that would justify the Precious One's decision to give him back his hat.

The same procession as before repeated itself then—the high Lamas led by the Debate Master, my dear mentor Geshe Lothar. The weather was sparkling clear, the sky a crystal blue, and the sun a glorious gold shining across the golden robes. It even bathed the Founding Father as he passed nearby, looking relaxed for once. And then came the two warriors.

Drom was his usual powerful presence, and even Di-di-la at his side looked bright and chipper. I guess it was the season, or the sun, or the knowledge that this was really the very last day of testing—or perhaps somehow everyone felt what was about to happen, I'll never know for sure.

Luckily Di-di-la came through on the left side, over close to me, and I was able at the last moment before he reached the gate to lunge through a few bystanders and thrust out my hand, with Tenzing's beads. Di-di-la looked over at me calmly, as if this were all part of the normal proceedings, and accepted the beads gracefully with both hands. Then he stopped right there in the middle of everything and slowly removed the old chipped beads from his own wrist and gave them to me, as Drom stood watching—not with a look of annoyance at the interruption, strangely, but with a sort of honest interest. And then they were on their way to that innocent little bench: the crucible in which Geshes were forged. The crowd and I settled down at the wall, to wait for the opening prayers to finish, and the Ancient One's hundred warriors took their seats on the timber platform behind the center wall.

"Excuse me, my lady."

I didn't even turn to see who was talking; "my lady" was reserved for women of nobility, and not country girls.

"My lady, Miss Friday? Niece to the Master Teacher himself?"

This time I turned, I suppose with a look of some astonishment, because the young monk at my side blushed and said, "Not to disturb you, my lady, but... but I have been sent by the Debate Master, who wishes that you would please come with me, if you would."

I felt a pang in my heart. So even Geshe Lothar was afraid to have me anywhere near the Founding Father. I shrugged and followed the young monk to the back of the crowd—no use ruining my obedient act before it even got started. Somewhere in the back there we were met by a chubby little novice about ten years old, carrying a bag almost bigger than he was.

From there the three of us did a wide circle through the fields and came around to the far side of the timber platform. The young monk had been given a stout oaken staff that served to identify him as an official from the monastery, and people made way for us as we threaded our way up to the front of the timbers.

We stopped there, right at the wall, and the young monk boosted himself up onto the platform. Then he turned and put his hand out to help me up. I was completely confused, and stopped there cold, like a mule.

"Please, my lady. Debate Master's orders, and this is his courtyard. Please."

I put out my hand and he pulled me up. I looked around and saw that this little corner of the platform had been roped off for special guests. Sitting there on big plush cushions were several noblemen and their ladies; no one I had ever seen, and I realized that they were probably patrons of the Ancient One's monastery, out to have a fine day in the country and enjoy the spectacle.

Right there in front of me was a very stuffy-looking matron with a daughter my age sitting on each side. They all had their hair done up the way that aristocratic ladies in our country used to wear it: their long lovely tresses coming up over the top of their heads on little wooden supports that looked like crowns, with the hair wrapped around and then studded with ornaments of red coral. Coral in our country was extremely rare and precious, since we are so far from the sea, and there was more of it loaded on each woman's head than I had seen in my entire life. They gave me a long stare, and then their eyes traveled across my worn-out farm dress and the bright country girl's apron. And then a moment later they were gazing back at the pavilion, satisfied that there was nothing more about me to see.

"Here please, my lady. Very specific, Geshe Lothar was very specific. Said you had to be right here," and the young monk motioned to the very front of the platform, where it met the opening for a gate into the courtyard. The gate itself was pushed open the other way, and monks were sitting up against the wood, but a small patch of courtyard had been left free, just inside the frame.

Then the monk waved to the little novice, who opened up his bag and handed up a big fine cushion, the kind that say a Chanting Master would sit on. My jaw dropped, and a little rustle went through the three Coral-Heads; big cushions are a big deal in our country. The monk arranged it neatly on the edge of the platform, right at the opening in the wall. Then he reached down to the novice and pulled up a fine golden seat cover: also normally reserved for, say, a monk who was already a Geshe. My jaw dropped further, and I was afraid to even glance at the expressions behind me.

The young monk didn't take any chances at that point; he fairly pushed me down on the cushion there and then came around to the front and said, "One more thing, my lady, if you please. Very specific he was, you see, and I know he'll check. So please, if only just to make my life easier; Geshe Lothar says specifically that you are to sit like the Loving One."

Now the Loving One, if you don't already know, is like a junior angel—that is, he's supposed to be the next Awakened One to show up in our world. And whereas almost all the other angels in pictures and such are sitting cross-legged, like everyone in Tibet and India does too—well, Loving One sits up on a chair the way people do in your western countries nowadays, with his feet down on the ground. This is all to signify that he's on his way here to our world, even as we speak.

And so to spare the young monk any trouble with the Debate Master, who I knew could also be a real taskmaster if he felt a young monk were shirking his duty, I pulled my dress around me and tucked it under and swung my feet down to the opening in the wall. And I looked down and saw that my toes, just the very tips of my toes, were actually *inside* the courtyard. The young monk leaned over and seemed to check on this very same thing, and then he straightened up and smiled and said, "Thank you, my lady," and jumped back down, melting into the crowd.

I glanced down gratefully at the chubby little novice; he gave me a big happy wink that I'm sure he'd learned from Geshe Lothar himself, and then he and his empty bag were gone too. I pulled my little lion out of his sling, and he settled comfortably into my lap, and we turned our eyes back to the battle.

42.

Angel Came Down

In that same moment that chanting suddenly stopped, and a hush descended it seemed over the whole earth itself. Even the song of the birds was still; even the wind held its breath. Di-di-la rose softly from his seat, clasping Tenzing's beads now between both his hands, and stepped out before the bench, to where the attacker must stand. He turned quietly, his tiny shoulders slumped and his head bowed low, and reached up to remove the corner of his monk's shawl, in the customary salute to his opponent. Drom nodded back gracefully, in a strange serenity that matched the mood of the whole world around us. Then Di-di-la raised his arm, his left arm, high into the air, thrusting Tenzing's beads to the sky. Every person there paused, and held their breath, and waited for the cry: the cry to battle, the sacred sound of wisdom, the sound of *Di!* My eye caught for a split second on the turquoise mother bead, hanging there in the blue of the sky, sparkling in the sun.

Di-di-la cried out *Di!* and in the same instant a golden bolt of sunlight seemed to strike the hand in the air, bursting down his body like lightning. He cried out again, a strange high cry that couldn't be a word, and his other hand flew up in the sky too; he lifted up high on his toes, and his head snapped back and his spine arched impossibly, as if someone had kicked him hard there, in the center of his back. His wide scared eyes spread ever so wider, staring at the sky in a kind of shock, like sockets in a skull.

And then suddenly he cried *Di!* again, leaping high into the air and whirling all the way around. *Di!* again, leaping to the left, past the front row of astonished senior monks. Then *Di-di!* and he had spun incredibly twice in the mid-air, dancing across the pavilion and vaulting over the opposite row of classmates, who as one raised their hands in an instinctive jerk to cover their heads. Then *Di-di-di!* with—was it six, or seven?—spins, maybe touching the ground, maybe not, flying past the judges on their three thrones. And then one last extraordinary leap, like a deer—one leg pointing ahead and the other pointing behind, his robes flying back in long golden streams—high into the air over the bench and Drom's head and hat, singing out *Di-di-di-di!* all the way.

424

And he landed somehow exactly as he'd started, facing Drom, both hands thrown high to the sky in joy, his head thrown back in exultation— and I could swear that for a split second he had beautiful long black hair flowing down past his shoulders, and bracelets of purest gold shining in the sun on his wrists, and instead of robes just the purest shimmering veils of golden silk floating down around his strong lovely slender golden figure: he was Gentle Voice, he was the Angel of Wisdom himself, and he sang out then, like a great bell, *"Di-di-di! I am Di-di-di! I am... Di-di-la!"*

I have to believe that Drom saw the same thing, because he sat on the bench transfixed, staring dumbfounded at little old Di-di-la. And Di-di-la—it was Di-di-la now, I guess—raised his eyes to Drom with the warmest smile I have ever seen and said in a loud clear friendly voice, "Now today, my brother, let us talk together... let us talk together, about kindness. *Kindness.*" And then he paused, and the silence around us was deafening. No one had even remembered to breathe again. Drom nodded, stunned, without a word.

"The Master, in his book on reasoning, starts out by saying that he has written the book only to help himself understand the subject more clearly, and not for anyone else's benefit. Now we clearly can't take that statement literally, can we? This is what I think he's really trying to say…" and Di-di-la, or whoever it was, went on like that—for two, three, four hours—leading Drom, and the rest of us, leading us by the hand, guiding us like a father would his beloved child through a lovely glade of green trees, with soft shafts of warm golden sunlight filtering in through the leaves, across a soft mossy path weaved between delicate, fragrant ferns.

It was not a battle—or like no battle the courtyard had ever witnessed—it was a symphony, it was the sound of gentle waves on the shore, it was the eloquence of silence itself. Drom sat perched upon the edge of the bench, very straight, his face in the bright beautiful smile of a happy child, as Di-di-la gently led him on, down the lovely paths of lovely ideas, holy ideas, ideas about kindness, ideas about goodness, ideas about compassion, all flowing one to the other, each one proving the next, each one establishing with the iron necessity of pure logic why every suffering living being on this planet should and must devote themselves to serving everyone else.

"My lady?" a voice shook me out of the trance of this most gentle war. I still wasn't used to the words ever being addressed to myself.

"My lady?" repeated the voice; it was a tall, thin novice of about fifteen years, calling up to the platform from among the crowd pressed happily to the wall, all in a trance of their own.

I automatically glanced behind me at the Coral-Head Trio to see which one he was talking to. They all had their heads turned demurely to the monk, as a My Lady should.

"My lady, Mistress Friday? Is there a Mistress Friday among you?" called the monk politely. The Coral-Heads looked around them, a bit confused, and then shook their heads.

"Uh... that... that would be me," I said a little nervously, raising my hand slightly.

"Oh yes," said the monk, "thank you." And he held his arm up high over the crowd and waved towards the back, and then before I knew it there were three more young monks clambering up onto the platform around Long-Life and I. One set a little wooden table down at my side—it was made of fine dark hardwood, carved into intricate figures of wild animals and fantastic eagles and dragons. The second monk whipped out a small green tablecloth of Indian brocade, covered the table, and set down there a beautiful wooden spoon, after making a great fuss about wiping it to a shine with a pure white linen napkin. And then the third monk carefully placed there a handmade silver bowl with a matching silver lid that had all kinds of silver filigree all over it. Then finally the tall thin one stepped up, positioned a lovely Chinese ceramic cup at just the right angle to the bowl, and poured out a fine golden tea from a small churn, which he then placed at the side of the table.

"Compliments of the Master Cook, my lady" he smiled then. "Says you'll understand. Careful of the bowl, now, it's a bit hot." I smiled back without any comprehension, and all four jumped back to the ground and disappeared among the people, who I noticed now were handing each other wooden bowls of hot tea, pushing them into each others' hands with odd huge smiles all over their faces. And they all stood there staring at Di-di-la strolling with Drom through the leafy glade of ideas, enjoying the warmth of the bowls in their hands as the evening chill began, completely forgetting to drink.

I waited respectfully for the grace to be sung by the Chanting Master and the assembled monks, even as Drom and Di-di-la continued their communion. And then I took a quick gulp of wonderful spiced tea and slowly raised the lid from the bowl.

And then I started to cry, right there under the glares of the Coral-Heads, pretty loud; I couldn't help it. Inside the bowl there was just a simple porridge, mixed with little orange slices of dried apricot and a kind of walnut we have, called *targa*. And maybe if you had been there you would have thought it looked rather ordinary. But in the courtyard, you see—among the warriors—this particular porridge is only served once a year, because it is the *geshe tukpa:* the Geshe's porridge, offered only to those who have just won their Geshe's hat.

43.

The Final Proof

I ate about half the Geshe porridge, just for
good luck—who could taste anything with the
delightful music emanating from the warriors?
Then with a naughty little smile to myself I set the
silver bowl with the rest of the porridge down on
the platform to my left, where the Coral-Heads
would be sure to see it, and let Long-Life down to
lap some of it up. This got a bit of a *hrrumph* from
behind me, and I was in such a good mood that I
held the exquisite teacup down and let Long-Life
have some too; then I raised it to my own lips and
gulped the rest. This got a gasp from all three. I
was considering fishing a piece of walnut out of the
leftovers—to hold it up so my little lion could get
up and do his prayers and then leap through the air
and grab the walnut in his mouth when I yelled
Bam!—but the "battle" was just too fascinating to

miss a moment more. Di-di-la was leaning towards Drom, with intensity.

"And so, you see, our habit of taking care only of ourselves—our habit of taking care only of what's on *this* side of the edge of our skin—it really is just a habit; and like any habit, we could with steady practice change it into a *different* habit: that is, we could train ourselves to see ourselves *bigger* than the edge of our own skins. Why, we could in time see ourselves stretch across the edge of other people's skins, and then we would take care of others just the way we take care of ourselves, because now our habit would be to *actually be inside them:* taking care of them *because* we take care of ourselves. And can you imagine what the world would be like if *everyone* picked up this new habit? Wouldn't it be *wonderful?*"

Drom let out a delighted giggle and gushed, "Why, I never thought of that!" Di-di-la paused with a happy smile and then took Drom's mind by the hand again and led him even deeper.

I chanced a glance at the three judges. The Abbot, the Precious One, was holding his own beads up to his heart happily, his head cocked to the side and his eyes fixed on the lovely being in front of Drom. The Ancient One was leaning back in his throne like a little kid, his hands down on either side of his hips, his entire face lit up with that big unabashed toothless grin. And the Founding Father, who in fact had been no mean warrior himself in his day, was leaning far over the front of his throne, straining to catch every nuance of Di-di-la's flow. Every once in a while, right after a crucial point had been made, he would snap back up straight again with a tremendous smile and a shake of his head, as if to say, "Amazing! Why, I never thought of that either!"

Then suddenly a call floated up from the crowd at my side: "My lady? Excuse me, my lady?"

I took a wicked peek at the Coral-Heads. They glared down at the monk and then all three very slowly raised their arms and pointed silently at me.

"Oh, yes—my lady, Mistress Friday?" It was a very handsome young monk whom I recognized from my trips to the scriptorium to collect the precious scraps of paper.

"I am Friday," I said, shyly, somewhat abashed.

He stood there squeezed between the dreamy-eyed spectators, pulled a shoulderbag around in front of him, and fished inside it for a moment. Then he took out a small package wrapped in a brilliant crimson cloth and handed it up to me with gentle respect.

"A gift," he called. "A gift for you from the Master Calligrapher, my lady. He said you'd understand."

I accepted the package with a look of surprise; the handsome young monk nodded with a pleasant smile, waved a little goodbye, and melted back into the crowd.

My hands were trembling; I set the gift in its precious cloth down on the lovely little table. Long-Life was curious and poked his nose at the package; he felt the energy coming from the thing, and I could fairly feel the breaths of the Coral-Heads down my neck as they too craned ahead to see what it was.

There was a silver-colored ribbon sewn to the cloth, and I unwrapped it slowly. The last fold of cloth slid off and there in my hands was an exquisite manuscript, all on fine parchment, with fresh calligraphy done in a true master's hand: each letter was like a work of art in itself. The top page said "The Three Foundations," and when I saw it I started to weep again. For this is a traditional collection of three of the Five Great Books into one volume, to make them easy to memorize. And it is a gift that is often made to a new Geshe, who together with his new hat has just earned the responsibility of passing the great books on to his own students.

I turned the page over and there, through my tears, I could see the line—the first line that Tenzing and I had ever heard: "Those who listen, seeking peace..." The tears burst out even stronger, and I heard a low murmur of sympathy escape from the lips of the ladies behind. I began to close and re-wrap the book and caught a glimpse of a little box drawn in the center of the first page of the first book. It was a custom to draw there the figure of some great teacher of the past; the caption below the box said, "Master Dharma Kirti." I smiled, because this was the very Master from ancient India whose book Di-di-la and Drom were travelling through now. It was an illustration of extraordinarily fine detail: this Lama is always drawn as a wisdom warrior, an attacker, with his hand held high, ready to come down in a tremendous clap, and a string of beads flying to the side from the wrist of his upstretched hand.

And then something more caught my eye, and I peered down. Beneath the Lama's tall hat were drawn a few thin lines, coming down the side of his face almost as though—instead of the close-cropped hair of a monk—he might have very long hair, perhaps tied back behind his head. And then I saw that his features were decidedly soft, nearly feminine, and that there was a low wall sketched in behind him, across the background. And the tiniest chip of turquoise had been glued there, into the beads flying from his hand.

It was no use crying even more. I just laughed and shook my head and looked up again to my brothers.

Suddenly the Debate Master stepped out to the front of the bench. My eyes, and a thousand others, broke away for a moment from Di-di-la. I, we all, looked around in amazement. The daylight was gone; no, it was in fact well into the night. Someone had come, and set out torches, and left. Bowls full of cold untouched tea were spread all over the top of the wall. And the night air was cold; freezing cold. Groggy people everywhere, monk and villager, were coming out of their trances and reaching to pull on cloaks and coats, to bundle themselves up.

Di-di-la had been standing well back away from the examination bench, guiding Drom and all the rest of us through a few final thoughts, like dessert after a wonderful meal. Every once in a while his hands came down in a clap that was nothing like a warrior's finger-splitter, more like a puff of fragrance or a pillow that left his palms and floated off to his opponent, as a kind of gift.

But now Di-di-la paused, and broke his eyes away from Drom's for the first time. Drom glanced around sleepily, like a child gently woken from a pleasant nap. Di-di-la glanced at Geshe Lothar and gave a brief, respectful nod, for stepping forward was the traditional signal that the Debate Master wanted the attacker to pose the final proof. And the proof in the final examination of a Geshe is always the same, even to this day.

Di-di-la straightened up, tall, as tall and mighty and graceful as any warrior who had ever stood in the courtyard. Then he approached Drom, slowly, and stopped only a foot or two away, as is the ancient custom for the final proof.

"There will never come a day," he said softly, "when every living creature upon this entire earth is freed from every form of pain, and even from death itself."

Drom's eyes, and his face, and his whole being gleamed in pure devotion. "Not so!" he called out powerfully.

"And why not?" called back Di-di-la, with the same power, tears bursting from his eyes, streaming down his cheeks.

"Because truth," and here Drom as well burst into tears, tears of total joy, "because truth is infinitely more powerful than all the illusions we live in. It must prevail. It will..." he cried, "... prevail!"

And Di-di-la bowed to Drom and to the truth, and then he sat down on the bench and put his arm around the big shoulders. There was not a sound, anywhere.

The Debate Master returned to the back of the bench, behind Drom. He set his hands there softly, on the same shoulders. He turned and raised his head proudly and looked to the three thrones.

The Precious One gazed down at the scene before him with a look of infinite tenderness and happiness, and he and all of us paused there for a long moment, to cherish what had passed, to remember it. And then he raised his hand, and held up his first two fingers. The Founding Father beamed, and nodded gently. The Ancient One touched two fingers to his forehead, in agreement and an ancient sign of respect. And so it was decided: second rank, a high honor, something to treasure for the whole rest of a life.

And then Geshe Lothar placed his hands ever so slowly upon Di-di-la's shoulders—those thin little shoulders, stooped over again like Di-di-la's, as the boy stared at the ground, almost looking nervous again. The Precious One cocked his head and cracked a big grin and held up one finger, very high, towards the stars. The Founding Father looked down at little Di-di-la, his eyes all soft and glazed over, still in the spell of the sacred thoughts the warriors had weaved that night, and nodded slowly, a single tear of happiness tracing its way down his iron features. And lastly the Ancient One just threw up his hands happily, as if to say, "Well, what else?"

There were no cheers. Custom was forgotten, and no one leapt up to wave their hat. Someone in the courtyard, someone up towards the front—I'll never know who—stood up silently. He bowed slowly towards the warriors, pressing his palms together in front of his heart—our age-old expression of respect and devotion. Then one by one other people stood and did the same, still in total silence.

And then everyone was up, and bowing, and I could hear people around me beginning to sob quietly, at the beauty, at the truth itself—the truth of kindness. The high Lamas came down off their thrones, and a path parted silently before them, out the courtyard, back to the gate in the great wall of the monastery. And last came the two warriors, arm in arm, crying and smiling.

Long Life and I went and shared a big warm hug with the three delighted Coral-Heads, and then I ran to find Uncle in the crowd.

44.

The Spell is Broken

We stepped on to the horse road, in the stream of villagers headed home, all of them speaking and looking at each other gently with a warmth I had never seen before. Uncle walked with his eyes fixed on the stars up ahead of us, still wrapped in all his golden ceremonial robes—for it was now quite cold. He had a look in his face of utter contentment and satisfaction over the final results of all his years of painstaking work with the young warriors.

At one point he just stopped and looked in my face and burst out happily, "Now *that's* what a *real* battle in the courtyard is supposed to look like!" And then he walked on silent and happy all the way home, never taking his eyes off the stars, as if he were just about ready to walk up and stay there among them forever.

We had a quick lunch the next day, and then left for the monastery as soon as two caravan women came to stay with Amala. One of them was Mutik, who would be the hostess for the Founding Father's dinner the next day. Uncle made sure I spent a little time with her, to talk and get acquainted; she was really quite nice—very bright and talkative, in a nice way—and I knew Uncle had made a wise decision, and felt better about it.

Uncle and I didn't say much on the way; we took the horse road, and it wasn't a hard walk, but the weather had turned back a bit towards winter, with strong winds funneling down the road between the trees on each side. Long-Life in the baby sling kept me warm in front, but Uncle and I both had trouble keeping our shawls up around our necks. After one particularly powerful gust Uncle laughed and said the leaves would probably be out early—we Tibetans say that the winds in early spring shake the trees and wake up their sap again, and that's why the leaves start. I looked off to the southwest, to the sky, because winds so strong usually meant heavy rains—but there was still no sign.

Uncle led the way through the monastery, and I followed like an obedient fifteen-year-old country girl who had never been there amongst the jumble of alleys and monks' rooms. We went up quite close to Geshe Lothar's and then turned left, towards the back of the monastery. On the way we ran into several small clusters of monks loaded down with white silk offering scarves and bags of roasted barley flour or nuts or dried fruits and other such presents that you might use to congratulate a new Geshe. The monks would spend the whole day this way, every one, going to visit friends or students who had passed the final test. Everywhere there were sounds of laughter and voices retelling the story of each battle fought—events growing ever larger, into monastery legends, with each passing hour.

Di-di-la's was up a flight of wobbly stone steps, in a row of three or four very small rooms above a longer building of monk's cells. From the top of the stairs I could see over the back wall of the monastery, right behind Di-di-la's, and off across the fields to the Great Western Forest. The wind up here was even stronger, and Uncle and I slipped gratefully into Di-di-la's tiny door.

He was sitting up against the back wall on a worn-out little cushion, with a small simple wooden table before him. This was piled high with silken scarves and about a dozen wooden bowls full of all kinds of little pastries and snacks— evidence of a steady stream of morning visitors. A middle-aged monk was seated next to him, talking excitedly about some amazing point that Di-di-la had made during the battle the night before; and Di-di-la was listening with a face that was obviously exhausted but also happy and very intent on the words, as though Di-di-la himself were hearing the point he'd made for the very first time.

"Ah! Master Teacher, sir!" exclaimed the older monk, and both he and Di-di-la jumped up to greet Uncle. "Extraordinary work you've done with these young warriors, Geshe Jampa Rabgay! Now I don't know if you know, but I've a young nephew who's just joined the monastery this month—really exceptional potential, despite the fact that he's a bit slow and perhaps lazy; but I was wondering, if you had some time to work with him…" and he pulled Uncle off to a corner as if to sell him an old tired horse. Uncle was too polite to escape, and so Di-di-la and I could enjoy a few words together.

We stepped to the opposite wall, which was covered with a complicated flow chart drawn in white chalk. It was common for an attacker to sketch out their plan of attack this way weeks ahead of a big debate, just to get off to a good start: there was no way to plan more than the first few exchanges, since you never knew which branch of a logical path the defender would choose to follow, and the possible combinations were hundreds.

"*Geshe* Di-di-la!" I exclaimed, with a huge smile. "Oh, I'm *sorry*, I mean… Geshe Di-di-la of the *First Rank!* Or rather, the *only* First Rank!"

Di-di-la blushed profoundly and put his hand up for me to stop.

"No, seriously, venerable Geshe. But I really have to ask. How did you do that? Where have you been hiding all that, all this time?"

Di-di-la looked me steadily in the eyes and said softly, "I really don't know, Friday... I honestly don't know. It was such a magical day to start with, and then... and then... when I held up my hand, with Tenzing's beads... well there was this flash, or a kind of jolt, like light, golden light, and it came down my back in a single flash, and then everything just changed, and all the words were singing in my mind, in a thousand voices, way up high, and all I did was just open my mouth, and let them all come out."

He put his hands behind him then and rubbed his back with a grimace. "And then, afterwards, well, everything just changed back again, and... well... now I feel tired and sore all over, as if a yak had been dancing on my back for a week! And people come and tell me stuff I said, and I can hardly remember it!

"Gosh! I hope they never ask me if I can d-d-do that again!" he smiled, with his eyes all big and funny, and we both laughed.

"Di-di-la, about the first battle, I don't know if you know…" I started.

"I heard everything from Uncle, later on," he said. "No need to ever talk about it again. We did the right thing in the end, my sister, and that's all that matters.

"I'm just worried that washing all those dishes will make my hands too soggy to clap any more," he laughed, holding out his hands. And then he saw Tenzing's beads there wrapped around his wrist and hastily started to pull them off. "Oh my! I f-f-forgot to give them back!"

I held my hand up. "Oh no, my honorable Geshe. I have nothing else to offer you today, and that's the best gift I can think of anyway. They surely belong with you. But you have to let me keep these!" I reached for the old string of beads around my neck, and Di-di-la nodded happily. Then he went to his little altar and pulled off a beautiful shining fifteen-foot long silk offering scarf that we call an *ashey;* one that is usually presented to a new Geshe by the Debate Master himself. Di-di-la placed it softly around my neck, glanced to see that the older monks weren't listening, and whispered simply, "Geshe."

I nodded gratefully and was afraid I would start crying, so instead I tried to say, in a cheerful voice, "So... when will you be coming out to help with the new School?"

"Why do you want t-t-to know?" laughed Di-di-la, breaking the tension.

"So I can save up a big pile of dirty dishes for you," I replied, only half in jest.

"We start right away," said Di-di-la earnestly. "Uncle told me he expects me there the day after tomorrow, in the evening. Told all of us not to come out tomorrow; something important going on, he said."

"Oh, yes," I replied, shivering a bit at the thought.

And then a shadow blocked the little doorway, and we both looked up. A tall figure in rich dark woolen robes ducked under, followed by a second one with huge shoulders that I would recognize in the dark. We stood face-to-face with Drom and the Founding Father.

Their faces had changed back, to what they had been before, or worse—to something even colder than they had ever been. The Founding Father laid his cruel eyes on mine for a single instant of utter disdain that seemed to scream out, "Nothing is forgotten"; and then he turned silently to fix Uncle with the same look. Uncle straightened slowly and met the eyes, without fear, and without the slightest trace of hatred in return.

"Master Teacher," nodded the Founding Father. Drom was silent. He glanced once towards my face, with a wordless insolence so strong that if I had been a man I think we would have fallen to blows with nothing more than that.

"Founding Father, sir," replied Uncle, and he gave a bow, the very low formal bow that is normally reserved for the Abbot himself. Going down Uncle caught my eye in a command that could be no clearer, and Di-di-la and I bowed as well.

The Father turned to Di-di-la, and stared down at the back of his neck for a moment, as if he longed to snatch up something heavy and break the thin little neck in two. And then a sort of a sigh came out of him, and he motioned to Drom, who extracted a short, tattered, yellowed offering scarf from his shoulderbag. He bowed to the Founding Father and made a great display of handing the scarf over with respect. The Founding Father took it and dropped it over Di-di-la's shoulders, as if he were shaking a rat off his hand. Then he snarled, "Congratulations," in a voice that said very loudly:

I have to do this, to maintain my image in this place, but please be sure I don't mean it at all.

"M-m-my... my humble thanks," squeaked Di-di-la. Then Drom reached out and thrust two old mushy apples in Di-di-la's hands, and there was a long moment of frigid silence. When we finally looked up, they were gone.

45.

Ten Minutes

That night the wind blew hard and cold, howling over the yurt, and I had strange dreams. At some point I was sitting with Grandmother and Amala and Tenzing, on the floor at the side of Uncle's bed, and he was repeating to me very carefully the instructions he had given to the young sage for his journey. I was trying very hard to remember them, but then I turned around and looked at the other three, and their faces were all haggard and pale as snow, and the fear of it woke me up. Towards morning I dreamt that I was a little girl again, laying under the covers next to Tenzing at the foot of the family fire, and it was all warm and happy and he was excited and telling me about a secret package he had seen behind Uncle's altar. But when I woke up it was all as cold and lonely as ever, except for little Long-Life asleep at my feet.

Just before noon, I heard someone come down the path from the horse road; it was Mutik, loaded with last-minute supplies. The wind was still gusting, and there were low dark clouds and a drop of rain now and again. I went out to take Uncle his lunch, knowing I would probably be exiled to my yurt after that.

"Ah, good!" said Uncle a bit nervously as I entered. "Good to get all our chores done and be ready before the guests come!"

I smiled cooperatively. I knew what Uncle was saying, and wanted him to know I knew. I also knew that the visit of the Founding Father was a very critical moment in Uncle's life, and in all our lives. If I thought about it, the happiness of many people, far into the future, depended on Uncle being free to carry out his plans. And so I had no intention of endangering them, and I wanted Uncle to know.

"That's right," I added brightly. "I thought I'd clean up after lunch and then go and study quietly in my room for the rest of the day. I can walk over to the family yurt and have a bite to eat with Amala at dinner, and then go back and do my usual stuff up to bedtime."

Uncle gave me a grateful grin. "Thanks, Geshe Friday. It's just this once, while people's emotions are still running so high. Then after that things will settle down and life I think will be quite exciting around here."

I nodded again to reassure this infinitely kind-hearted man, and went to the door. Uncle leaned out over his bed and took a long look at the sky through the doorway; his face seemed rather worried. A few hours later he was at my own door, all bundled up against the cold and the wet.

"Friday," he said sharply. "I've got to be going. Should have left hours ago. It's really not right for the Founding Father to be walking all the way out here in this kind of weather without an escort; it might get dark early, he might mistake the way, anything could happen."

"But Drom knows the way very well," I said, with no wish to see Uncle out in the weather himself.

"Oh yes... I know... but really, what occurred to me," said Uncle, sounding a little out of breath, "was that... if I go... if I go myself all that way, well then... the Father will know, he will know that I really want to be reconciled with him. Do you see?"

I gazed at Uncle in wonder. You see, in our country a Lama is being very humble if he goes a long way to escort another Lama to his home, especially if the weather is bad—it's a very clear way of saying, "You are so much greater than me, and I am so honored to have you come to my place." And in my mind one Uncle was worth a thousand Founding Fathers. But I also realized that it was Uncle's very humility that made it so.

"I do see, Uncle. Please take care." I knew he'd be going by the back way, over the slate ridge, to save a lot of time—and in the rain it was particularly treacherous.

"Oh yes, of course. I... I mean, it will be all right, I'm sure." I smiled again. Uncle never said anything more about his special abilities than that. "And don't worry about Mutik at all," he went on, in a hurry. "She has absolutely everything she needs, and I've asked her not to leave the school yurt at all. It must be toasty warm and floating in delicious smells from now until the moment we arrive."

I nodded again, and there was a strange moment between us. I looked into his eyes, the old kind sad eyes, and he looked into mine, with a tenderness; and then he nodded silently, and glanced to the floor, and was gone.

I went back to writing out the most complicated letters of the Mother Tongue for about the fiftieth time that day, but it was cold and Long-Life was bored and I finally got up to stretch my legs. I wanted to make a fire in the pit but I knew that Uncle would be bringing the Founding Father in along the horse road and down the path right past my door—and so better I guessed if it looked like I wasn't home at all, or like I just didn't exist altogether. So I stretched a bit and then started doing some of Uncle's special movements, and Long-Life perked up and stretched himself a bit on the bed too, and I laughed and then tripped over my long dress one more time. It really does get in the way, I thought, as I sat on the floor nursing a bump on my bottom. If I could only get a good look at Uncle's white loincloth, I could put one together for myself in about ten minutes.

Just ten minutes.

But he's never gone.

But he's gone now.

Not today.

When, tomorrow? When Di-di-la's around 24 hours a day? When fifty villagers are coming and going for lessons every day?

Just ten minutes.

Yes, just that—just ten.

But where does he keep it?

Tenzing. The dream. "Uncle has a secret," behind the altar, behind a stone, a stone that comes out.

I stood there and thought furiously. I knew I would never have another chance. I knew it was wrong, but I knew it was important, very important, like a child making the *zadak* alarm, a child who was not supposed to.

And I knew too that there was no way Uncle and his cruel guests could ever show up in less than two or three hours. If there was to be a time, it was only now.

I threw on a shawl and went out into the cold, Long-Life at my side; a steady rain had started, struggling down between gusts of wind that threw the branches of the trees, and flattened the grass, and blew anything loose around the yurts and the clearing with cold slaps and clangs.

I walked as I knew Grandmother would have: striding with confidence and my head up, as if I had real business to do in Uncle's yurt and went in it regularly when he was out. But Mutik was nowhere to be seen; smoke whipped out the sky window of the school yurt, and I knew she was occupied.

I stepped up to Uncle's door and put my hand to the latch. We didn't have locks or anything like that in those days; if a person went out, they simply closed the latch on their yurt door, and anyone who came to visit them saw the latch was closed, knew they were out, and just came back later. I knew some monks who would even have someone else latch their door from the outside every morning, so they could pray and do their meditations all day, and no one would guess they were home or even bother to knock. I knew that lifting the latch was the point from which I could not return, and I hesitated, but only for a moment.

Uncle's yurt was full of warmth and light even in the miserable weather. I felt a kind of reverence there, especially now, by myself—as though I had entered a very lovely chapel. I went to the altar and looked down at the beautiful bowls of water and the small, carefully tended figurines of all kinds of angels and holy beings. Then my eyes went to the wall, and with a deep feeling of satisfaction I saw hanging there the tapestry I had so carefully woven—the exquisite letters of the Mother Tongue. And then I stooped down and wormed my arm and shoulder back behind the altar; Long-Life too pushed his little chest in curiously, anxious to help me, as always.

It took a while to find the stone, and my fingers were trembling a bit as I began to imagine Uncle having forgotten something, and walking back in, and finding the new obedient me there being the least obedient ever. But finally a stone moved, and I slid it out, and there underneath was a very ordinary white cotton cloth, wrapped around a small package.

It felt right, and I was too scared to open it there. I went out and latched the door carefully and did my Grandmother walk across the clearing again, but nobody was looking. Dusk was indeed falling very early, and the rain was pelting down.

Long-Life and I got back to our room; it was nearly as cold inside as out, and it made my hands tremble all the worse. I sat down on my bed and put the white package in my lap and opened it carefully, Long-Life peering up over my thigh.

Inside on top was a tiny little book, not more than ten or twenty leaves of a very old parchment, covered in careful, minute strokes of the Mother Tongue. The letters were a little different from the ones Uncle had shown me, and I knew they must be very old—I could still make most of them out, although I had no idea what they said. And then below that lay the sacred cord.

I pulled it out carefully, still expecting Uncle to sweep in any moment, not with anger but worse—with his trust in me broken. The wind had gotten even stronger, turning the yurt into a little symphony of sharp noises—window flap flying up and down, roof poles squeaking and groaning, lashes of rain sounds tearing across the walls—and my heart jumped with each sound, thinking Uncle was at the door.

But the cord—it was so soft, so beautiful, so special—Uncle's warmth pouring out of it, lovely crimson threads twisted amongst the white. I held it for a long while and then took out the loincloth, which I saw now was really just a long piece of very worn, soft white cotton, radiating with Uncle's energy, with years of dedicated practice. I stood up and got a measuring stick and bent down to get the size just right, knowing I could have it safely back to Uncle's now in a matter of minutes.

And as I stood there I heard a voice. It was a woman's voice, the voice of an older woman, and for a split second I thought it was Grandmother. But it wasn't. It was someone else, someone I had never met—yet.

And she said, strongly, "Put it on."

I froze. I even glanced around. But there was no one. I hesitated.

"Put it on, *now*. It's important."

The silence came upon me. I couldn't really do anything else. I was just watching myself, and I was starting to put on the sage's cloth. I took off my dress and my blouse and set them quietly on the bed next to the holy little white package. I picked up the cord as if I had picked it up every morning of my life and set it in its familiar place, there on my shoulder. And then I picked up the loincloth and wrapped it around and under and tucked it back in with the quick, unthinking motion of years of practice.

It was cold, despite the burning heat of the cloth. But I couldn't make a fire. I went to the altar and took out all the little butter-lamp cups I had—six or seven—and set them together in a row, and lit them.

A warmth and a golden light, like a little piece of sun, filled half of the yurt, from floor to ceiling. The loincloth called to me: Let us dance, as we have danced forever. And I heard it, and put my palms together in silent happiness, and reached them to the sky, to the glorious golden light of the Sun, with all the joy I have ever known. And we held there, silent, still, for it seemed beyond all time.

And then suddenly there was a tremendous gust of wind and rain, and it threw the window flap up against the top of the yurt and held it there, slapped it there hard, for a full minute. And in that time I stood, frozen in that glorious golden light, and turned my eyes out to the gloom of the early dusk. And there I saw the Founding Father, and Drom, standing motionless on the path, each holding the reins of a horse behind him. And they were staring in at me, staring with all their might at the bare-chested girl in the sage's cloth, in the sage's dance. And then the wind's hand let go the window flap, and it fell, and the hopes of my whole life fell with it.

46.

My Little Geshe

I dropped to my knees and stayed there, on all fours, my heart beating wildly. Then I crawled to the window and peeked out between the flap and the wall. The Founding Father and Drom had walked on a bit towards the school yurt, still leading their horses. Drom had his back to me and was looking intently into the face of the Founding Father before him. And that face—those eyes—held a look of glee, a very evil kind of glee; the Father was still staring towards my yurt but with a look of exultation, of impending victory. His hand was raised up in the air in excitement as he spoke to the young man, and then suddenly he made several sharp chopping motions with it, and waved in a wide arc around at the whole homestead. And then Drom said something—a question—and the Founding Father smiled and slowly shook his head, turning his hand in a circle, as if to say: Tomorrow.

And then Mutik was bounding out the door with a gracious smile, bowing low and waving the visitors in out of the rain. They tied up their horses and I heard little pieces of sweet oily pleasantries from the Father to Mutik: "Decided to come out a bit early... avoid the rain, such a trouble you know... rode the horses to make better time... pleased to be here, very pleased; you'd never guess how pleased." And then they all stepped into the school yurt.

I crawled back and sat in front of the altar, my heart hurting now in some kind of dull pain. Somehow, in a few minutes' time, I had managed to ruin everything which that noble man—my Uncle—had spent a lifetime to build. No, worse: it could even be his life at stake now, when the Founding Father got back to the monastery, and called the Council, and described how this secret sage was still corrupting young people, young women, with the arts of healing that no one understood, and many might misunderstand. And in the process of eliminating Uncle, whose work with his nephew was finished, the Father would smash and disgrace our family too. I stared dumbly at the stones of the altar. It was all ended, and there was nothing I could do.

And then Long-Life came, and put his paws up on my lap. He looked up to me with eyes that looked almost human—sad eyes, sad for me. But eyes that were saying something too. And then I saw that he had the red baby sling in his mouth.

I pulled them both up on my lap and stroked Long-Life's luxurious hair; it calmed me, and thoughts began to form themselves in my mind, one by one.

First, there was no doubt that the Founding Father would wait; he would wait here, at the homestead. Mutik would tell him Uncle had gone to escort him and that he'd be back soon—my guess was that it would be about an hour, once Uncle knew that he had missed the Father. And the Founding Father would enjoy an exquisite last meal with Uncle, without saying a word about what he had seen, and then in the morning my father would return from caravan, and there would be a long cordial meeting, and the Founding Father would extract promises of every single penny he could get. And then, only then, he would return to the monastery, and call the Council, and force even the Precious One to destroy this pure and innocent man.

And there was nothing I could do: there was no way to take back what the Founding Father and Drom had both seen; no way to stop them from believing that Uncle was teaching me the sage's way as well as the Geshe's, and that he had given me the sacred cloth and cord.

Long-Life stirred in my lap. The red wool strap of the bag was still in his mouth. He dropped it into my hand. I fingered the soft wool thoughtfully, and then it all came clear.

What if someone else had given me the loincloth? What if Uncle himself had no sage's cloth? What if I took all this trouble upon myself, and took it away, for good? I clasped the red bag tight in my hand. Yes, that was the right way, and it would save everything.

I got up quickly and reached for my blouse and dress, pulling them on over the cord and the cloth. There was no way I could get them back to Uncle's, and I knew that the Founding Father had enough authority to order a search of any monk's room—even that of a monk who was living outside the monastery.

I gazed around the yurt once, slowly, thinking very clearly now. I would need some good shoes, and something to stay a little warm, if not dry. I rummaged through Grandmother's chests quickly and found just what I was looking for: her old Northerner's boots, made of a thick gray felt that came up all the way to the knees. I sat down and pulled them on; they were tight, but it would have to do—there was no time, I could not risk running into Uncle. And then there was a very thick, woolen, dark red shawl, much larger and warmer than the one I had used back in the days of the lady with the baby. Was it only a few weeks ago? I shook my head. It was centuries ago—it belonged to a past that was leaving today, and would never come back.

I went to the altar and stood there for a few minutes, gazing at all the things with love, thinking of Grandmother Tara. It felt right to have her clothes on me at this moment, and again I thought she would have been proud.

I grabbed her little red pouch of dried cheese, and the Calligraphy Master's book, and then Uncle's little parchment too. I stood and thought for another moment and then got the Geshe hat out, and stuffed everything hurriedly into the baby sling, along with the long white greeting scarf that Di-di-la had given me—was it only yesterday?—but that past was leaving now quickly too.

I threw the sling over my shoulder. I stooped and picked up Long-Life in one arm, then took my pillow with the other hand. If the Founding Father got my room searched too, they would find nothing that a *girl* wasn't supposed to have. I blew out the butterlamps and stood there for a minute in the dark, my insides beginning to churn. And I left.

Outside I stooped and cut to the right, back behind the cover of my yurt—but it was almost completely dark anyway, and the rain coming down hard. I ran and slipped into the door of the family yurt; here it was almost completely dark too, only the last embers of a fire glowing in the pit, and a single butterlamp burning on the altar. Amala was sitting up in bed, with the covers over her legs, staring down at the blanket intently, picking little threads off of it. She didn't even look up when I came in.

I glanced at her with a torn heart and then moved quickly, so I wouldn't have time to think about it. I pulled a water bag of Father's off the wall and filled it from a pitcher. I got out his parchment and bamboo pen, sat down, and carefully wrote out two notes. Then I wrote out a small slip of parchment that said, "for Geshe Di-di-la," slid it under the front fold of the Master Calligrapher's precious little book, and placed it on the altar. And last I went to sit on the bed, close to Amala, facing her. I pushed my pillow with its years of tiny scraps of writing behind her thin, fragile back. Surely not even the Founding Father could disturb this crippled soul.

"Amala," I said, my voice and my heart cracking. She still didn't look up, hands picking nervously at the threads. I didn't know if she could even hear what I had to say, but I had to say it.

"Amala, I love you so much…" I started to cry. I took her hand. It was soft and warm. She still didn't look up.

"Amala, I have to go… I have to go away, for… for a while." The sobs came up and stopped me. She didn't look up.

"I am going… I am going, because it will help everybody else, and…" I gazed sadly at the dark stones of the floor, where my brother used to lie warm and happy, next to me. "…And because I need to find something out; I need to learn something, something that will help you, something that could have helped Grandmother and Tenzing—I need to learn the healing, all of it. And when I do, I will come back, I will come back for you… I swear it." I wept again, quietly, the tears falling on our hands. Amala stared down at the tears, motionless.

When I could, I looked up at her again and said, "And there is something you must keep for me; it is something I worked very hard to get for you, because you wanted it so much, and because… because I love you so very much." I pulled out the cloth with my Geshe hat inside, and placed it in Amala's lap, and opened it.

Her eyes went to the hat. She set her hand softly on top of it and felt its worn softness. And then I saw a single tear fall on the gold of the hat, saw the little droplet melt very slowly into the fabric of it.

And then Amala straightened up, and looked me straight in the eyes, and opened her mouth. And her tongue twitched and a dry rasping sound came up out of her throat, and it said, "My... little... Geshe." And she took me in her arms, and pulled my head to her chest, and held me there while I cried. Then she gently let me go, and looked at me again, and nodded, and I was gone.

47.

Inside the Lady of Freedom

I went quickly to the stone shrine, took Di-di-la's scarf out of the sling, and tied one end of it to the stones at the edge, about waist high. Then I took the other end and tied it to one of the poles of the cattle pen, so that the scarf stretched across the back path, the one that came in from the ridge—for Uncle would surely be returning this way. Then I stooped and reached back into the little archway, pulled out three butter lamps, and lit them, keeping them far back out of the wind and rain. And then I put my hands around the lovely bronze statue of Tara, the Lady of Freedom, and pulled her towards me a bit. I set her carefully on her back and pried off the little cover at the bottom of the statue. This is sort of a secret little compartment that our craftsmen always leave there, so you can stuff your favorite little holy things like special pebbles or a shell or a few pages of prayers inside of the Angel, and you always know where they are. Then I took Uncle's precious little book out of the baby sling, rolled the pages up tight into a cylinder, and slid them inside—they just fit. I tapped the cover back on with a stone, and put the Lady back in her place.

And then last I took out one of the letters I'd written, and propped it there between the statue and the stones. On the outside I'd written *Zadak—Danger!* in big red letters; I stepped back down the path a few yards and checked. It was perfect. From this angle the lights were bright, and the letter called out to be read. No one could miss the scarf. And none of it could be seen from the homestead.

This is what I wrote to my dear Uncle, not knowing if I would ever see him again:

Dear Uncle Jampa:

Something very bad has happened. The Founding Father and Drom came early, and through my window they saw me doing movements like a sage, in a white loincloth that I picked up somewhere. I'm afraid they will think that you gave me the cloth, and that you taught me the moves they saw, and I know this could cause a lot of serious problems.

And so I am leaving, I am going to India, because I really want to learn how to help people heal themselves. I beg you not to try to find me. You and Di-di-la must go on with the teaching you have planned; it is so important for so many people.

Please tell Father everything that has happened, and that I love him very much — that I will make him very proud, and that I will be back to Amala and him when I have learned what I must learn. I know that the caravan women will go on helping with the weaving, and that Di-di-la will serve you well, so I'm not worried about the family.

Please know that, by the time you read this, monks at the monastery will have been told that the young thread sage who traveled through a few months back was teaching me secretly, and that I have run away with him to his place in the Eastern Provinces. Drom and his friends saw me with him at the courtyard, as did Geshe Lothar, and everyone will remember.

*In a way it almost seems that
things will end up even better this way; I
think you see that too. Please pray for me,
and send me your blessings, and know
that no one could ever have been as kind
to me as you have. I hope that what I
learn will repay that kindness, always—
and I love you so very much.*

Your devoted niece,
Friday

*PS: My friend Dolma has the book
of prayers you loaned me from your altar.
The rest I had to take with me.*

I went over each word of the letter in my
mind, carefully. There was nothing that could
cause Uncle any more trouble if someone else
should see it. "Dolma" is a common girl's name in
Tibet; it is also our word for Tara, the Lady of
Freedom. I knew Uncle would know where to find
his little sage's book, when things had settled
down.

I took one last fond look at the Lady, in the
shining of the lights. Then I scooped up Long-Life,
set him in the sling, and covered us both as well as
I could with the shawl. We crossed quickly back
around the family yurt, and then walked through
the brush near the path to the horse road. The ridge

path would be quicker to the monastery, but there would be no way to avoid meeting Uncle on his way back, and I knew that must not be. This kind man would make me stay, and sacrifice himself to the Founding Father.

I knew too that we had to stay clear of the horse road—there was always a chance that someone would see me headed towards the monastery, and report it later—and anyway, the way would be a river of mud by now; far too slow. And so Long-Life and I started straight out across the fields and open country, running parallel to the road. It would be difficult going with patches of deep mud, but not nearly as bad as the road.

That walk I don't remember much. I cried a lot of the way, but it didn't matter—the rain was whipping across my face with the wind; my hair was catching everywhere around my throat, in my mouth as I gasped, under the strap of the bag. I just let it go. Sometimes I ran, as far as I could, and then other times I was slipping and falling on stones, among the sharp bushes, trying to protect Long-Life with my arms. The rain pierced the shawl and my dress as if they were not even there—I ran, I pushed myself on, like a mad woman, naked to the elements.

The monastery wall came up on me suddenly: my head was down, choking for breath, with steam pouring out of my lungs like a horse in winter. I was shaking all over from the wet and the cold, and I could feel Long-Life's little body trembling against mine too.

The main gates were of course closed and barred for the night; I'd known they would be, and I also knew where our only chance was. We circled around to the courtyard side, close to the wall. We stopped about ten feet from the smaller side gate, and stood there, flat up against the great wall, as unmoving as the stones. Rain flew into my face, and leaked off the wall down my back. I wasn't really thinking any more. I just stared off into the dark, and the dark fields, and told myself that I was made of stone, as patient and as still as the stone, until the moment came.

And then later—maybe it was an hour, or two, I don't know—the winds let up for a few moments, and there was a gap in the rainclouds: I could even see a few faint stars. And there was a noise at the gate that went through the wall and into my back. I came back to myself. Someone was taking the bar from the gate.

I looked up at the sky and held my breath, and pressed into the wall as far as I could. I heard the gate swing on its hinges, and then saw a thin, hunched-over figure step out. He moved with the look of an old man, shuffling out into the field and mumbling as he went. He stooped down there and began to relieve himself.

I kept my eyes on his back and crept sideways, still flat against the wall. Then suddenly he was finished and stood up, straightening back his robes. And so I simply ran the last few steps, slipping into the shadows of the open archway just as he turned around.

Inside I kept again close to the wall, circling around towards the back of the monks' rooms. I pulled the shawl up over my head and down my front as far as I could. In some places we had to cut across porches or down little alleys with windows close in on each side. But everything was boarded shut against the storm, and there were very few candles going. I knew then that it must be very late. No one was up chanting any books at all, and there was only the sound of a single handbell, far away— someone using the energy of the storm and the silent hours to make an offering of song to the Awakened Ones.

I came to the back gate of the wall then and knew where I was. I turned inside between two buildings and saw the old stairway. I climbed carefully to the top—the rain and wind were back again, with a fury, nearly knocking me off. There was a moment of confusion and fear while I tried to remember which door it was. And then I tapped, urgently, on the wood, praying that Di-di-la would hear.

The door opened slowly then, and Di-di-la looked up at me, half asleep. I dropped the shawl from my head, and his big funny eyes opened up wide as saucers.

"F... F... Friday! Friday! Oh my g-g-goodness. What are you doing here? What are you doing?"

I glanced over his shoulders and pleaded with my eyes. He hesitated a moment, and poked his head out and took a quick look each way, then pulled me inside and shut the door in an instant. Then he whirled around and stepped up to me with a look of concern, almost anger.

48.

End of the Lapdog Days

"F-F-Friday! What?" he hissed. "Now this is t-t-too much! What can you possibly be doing here, in the middle of the night, in the middle of this storm? You... you'll get me thrown out of the monastery forever!"

I tried to open my mouth to explain, but I couldn't move it right—my teeth were chattering, and my lips were all numb, and I just started to cry again, in relief to be with him, in fear of what would come.

"Oh m-m-my," he said then, really looking at all of me for the first time. "Oh my. Oh Friday, look at you... soaked to the bone. I'm sorry. Come, come sit down." He helped me get the sling off, and we set poor little Long-Life on the bed, and Di-

di-la covered him with his threadbare little blanket. Then he sat me down there next to Long-Life, and looked around helplessly for something to wrap me in, and finally got up and pulled his monk's shawl off his little stool and spread it over my shoulders. "What the heck!" he said cheerfully. "If I'm going to get caught with a girl in my room, might as well have her dressed up in my robes too!"

I laughed a bit and felt better, and Di-di-la pulled out the small tea churn that is as much a part of a monk's room as his altar, and poured me some tea into a small wooden bowl. I took a few gulps and then coughed for a bit, trying to stifle the sound with my fist. I realized I was still sick from the night at the first battle in the courtyard—so very long ago, so very far away, and I felt the heat of a fever already coming on. Di-di-la waited patiently, with courage to wait like that. And then I turned to look into his kind face, my new brother's face, the face of the second brother I was to lose.

"Di-di-la... Geshe Di-di-la. Something very bad has happened. I... I don't have time to tell you everything. I don't know if you really know why I wanted so much to study what you and Tenzing were studying.

"It was all because of my grandmother, and then later Tenzing—I had heard about the Wheel of Life, I had heard that what the Geshes learn can stop the Lord of Death, and so... and so I tried, I tried so hard. And it has made me ready...

"And now that I have learned those things... I have learned enough to know, to know that there is a part of it all that the thread sages keep, and so now if I really want to learn to help people—to help them heal themselves, I mean—I know I must learn the way of the sages.

"And I was playing around today in my room, wearing a sage's cloth that I had gotten ahold of... and the Founding Father and Drom... they came to the homestead, they came too early, and they saw me, through my window...

"And I'm afraid they will find a way to blame Uncle, and do something very bad to him, and ruin all the plans you both have to help others..." I stopped for a moment and stared down at the bed. Di-di-la was silent; I could feel his compassion for me, pressing against me like the wind outside.

I looked up at him; I knew it must go quickly now. "I can't tell you more... and it's enough... you see, you see what there is. I have something here—I need your help; and then I think things will be all right."

I reached for the baby sling and found the parchment inside. Miraculously it was dry; I realized that Long-Life had been covering it the whole way. I held it in the palms of my hands for a moment, and then I brought my eyes up intensely to Di-di-la's.

"This is a letter that I've written. It's to you, but in the morning—very early, just as people are getting up for the dawn prayers in the temple—you must go and show it to the Debate Master, to Geshe Lothar.

"And when he has read it you must tell him to go quickly and show it to the Precious One, the Abbot. Tell him I said, tell him Friday said, that the Abbot must see the letter immediately—it is very important, it could be a matter of life and death.

"You don't need to say exactly when or how you got the letter, I'm not asking you to lie for me—I would not put you in a position like that again..." I sighed and handed him the letter. "Please read it."

Di-di-la opened the parchment, and bent his head, and read.

My dear friend Di-di-la:

I writing you this leter tell you I leaving home, I running away with young thread sage you all saw me with before, at the courtyard. I fall in love with him then, and he gived me a white sage cloth, and teached me some, which no one else want to do. And now today he come back for me, and we go to his place in Eastern Provinces. I am saying you goodby, and asking you please help my famly much as you can.

With big thank-you,
Friday

When he had finished Di-di-la sat silently for a moment, staring down at the letter in his hands. Then he raised his head and looked at me with a kind of pain, his eyes brimming with tears.

"It is not t-t-true," he said. "You are covering something; you are protecting… you are taking something on yourself…" He said it as a statement, not as a question.

I looked down again, and then said softly. "You Geshes… you Geshes… you know too much, you figure out too much." He smiled through his tears.

"I will not tell you more," I said. "I will not have you lie for me, if they ask you whether you know anything else. But... but do you think it will work?"

Di-di-la grinned again, but I could see that his lips were trembling with emotion. "It will work... yes, I'm afraid it will work. Everybody... everybody is ready t-t-to believe that a girl like you is ready to run away f-f-for romance. Nobody is ready to believe that you have mastered the knowledge of a Geshe, and that you seek to know the sage's ways, s-s-so you can p-p-put them both together and learn how to heal people, to stop the Lord of Death." He paused for a moment, and I spent the moment, that last moment, to look at him, to love him, to know that he truly understood what I was doing, to know that he was a true brother, a brother of the heart.

"And I must say," he said finally, smearing a stream of tears across his cheek with the back of his hand, "I must say that it's brilliant. It saves... it saves everyone. And you c-c-can learn what you need to learn, and still come back any day you want, because n-n-no one will blame a young girl who was practically k-k-kidnapped by a thread sage. I, I especially like the atrocious spelling and grammar—obviously written by a s-s-simple girl— and no one can accuse... anyone else... of helping you write it." He stopped, and cleared his throat, and then added softly: "And you... you will... you are... coming back?"

I looked him again in the eyes, so he would know that what I would say next was true. "Di-di-la... brother... I am leaving because... because I must come back. I am leaving... everything, everyone that I love... because I love them, because I must learn how to really help them. We... we cannot go on like this, we... we cannot go on like before, people getting sick, people dying, people sitting in the darkness of a yurt mourning for those who died, until they die themselves—people trying to help people having to live in fear, in fear of people who refuse to help people. It's crazy, it's wrong. I will be back, I must come back—I will bring back what I learn, I will bring back the healing, and we... we will stop, we will stop all these things, these very wrong things."

Di-di-la nodded simply. The tears were pouring all over now, like the rain. I got up. We put Long-Life back in the sling. I took my brother's hands and bowed my head to him. He nodded and bowed his to mine, and our foreheads touched in the ancient way. And perhaps there was a little flash of gold that came down my back, from where his head touched mine—or perhaps I just imagined it. I turned and ran to the door, and left.

The rain was harder, and the wind, if that was possible. I came down the stairs clinging to the side of the building, and went to the back gate of the great wall. I lifted up the bar and stepped up to the threshold. Before me it was only darkness—the howling of the wind, throwing rain into my eyes, and the night, and the dark expanse of the monastery fields, empty from winter, a sea of mud stretching to the edge of the Great Forest.

I paused. The roads to India, the roads south, lay to my left. If Father or Uncle tried to find me, and I knew they would, they would be combing those roads. If the Founding Father—or anyone else from the monastery—cared to search for me and the young sage, they would send people out on the roads to the east, out the front gate of the monastery. And that was all as it should be, because Long-Life and I, we were going this way; we were going west, to the Great Forest, and then... to Katrin. *Katrin*—the name of the Master Sage sang in my heart, the way it had sung from the first moment I'd heard it. We would go to Katrin, we would find him, find him somehow, and he would teach me the rest of the healing.

I turned and pulled the gate tight, and took—took, I think it was, four steps into the field. And then I realized that I could just go north too, just walk up towards the slate ridge, and be home, in a couple of hours. And it would be warm and

Uncle would give me some tea and put me to bed, and in the morning he and Father would work things out with the Founding Father. And in time I could learn a lot from Uncle, if not everything...

Suddenly Long-Life went wild. He jolted and scratched and fought his way up out of the sling, and before I could stop him he leaped out into the air. He came down hard in the mud, one little front leg bent under him wrong, and he fell on his side and lay there for a second. I was stunned—I couldn't move to help him.

And then he got up slowly, and raised his head, raised it to the Western Forest. The whole side of his face, and his little body, were covered in mud. His luxurious hair was plastered against him, the beautiful fan of his tail was dragging filthy through the water. He walked ahead, into the field, limping a bit on the leg. But his head was raised, raised proud, ahead.

And when he had gone a few yards he turned his head, and looked back at me, looked back at me with a fire that killed the cold. "The lapdog days are over," said his eyes, "over, for both of us. This is what we are now; and it is hard, and it is going to be hard."

Then he turned back and walked straight on to the Forest, and never once did he look back, to see that I was following.

49.

The Inbetween

I remember crossing the fields—the sound of Grandmother's boots sucking out of the mud with each step, and the cold of rainwater seeping in around my feet, and the dark outline of the Great Forest ahead of us, illuminated by occasional flashes of lightning. And then after that we were only among the high black shapes of the trees, and the mud gave way to a slick silent carpet of pine needles. My mind was dead from exhaustion, and the empty vacuum into which my life had suddenly been thrown.

It was Long-Life who saved us; the new Long-Life, a wild silent determined thing moving steadily through the dark. My tired eyes kept the little patch of white always just in sight, forcing my legs to move exactly as much as needed, ignoring my mind. He walked; I followed, thoughtless.

At some point the rain began to slow, and then later it began to get much colder, and I knew that dawn was close now. A few minutes later I almost stepped on Long-Life, stopped in a soft flat spot within a circle of five ancient, gnarled trees. He was looking up at me in sheer exhaustion, his tongue falling out the side of his mouth and the injured leg bent halfway into the air, as if he could no longer even bear to stand on it. And I fell down on my knees, and then laid down, gathered his precious warmth into my arms, and fell asleep.

It was already afternoon by the time I awoke, my forehead now fiery hot from the fever, and the bones in my back and legs full of pain. I sat up in a soft column of sunlight coming straight down between the trees, and saw my little lion a few feet away on the bed of grass, sitting up very straight and alert, scanning the forest around us. And when he saw I had awoken he came to me slowly, limping slightly, and nuzzled against my cheek, as if to take away some of the heat.

I coughed a bit, and got out Father's water bag, and we both drank greedily, although we were still damp from the night before. Then I pulled out Grandmother's little red bag, with the little squares of dried cheese, and just the feel of it—something that had been a comfort all of my childhood, almost the last remnant of my childhood now—brought new comfort to us both. We chewed in silence for a long time; I scratched Long-Life behind the ears absent-mindedly and stared at the newness of the forest around us. I carefully avoided the gaping hole of loneliness and doubt so close at mind. And Long-life felt it too and got up decisively and walked to the edge of the clearing, looking back once to tell me we had to move on now, while we still had daylight.

The rest of that first day was much like the night before; my mind was still numb from all that had happened, events all just a blur now, along with a dim awareness of growing worry back at home—Uncle and Father's thoughts calling out for me, brushing me even here. And with the tiredness came then doubts about what I was doing, themselves more exhausting than anything else.

But Long-Life wisely left me no time to think on things much; the trees around us grew tighter and darker, and the ground began to slope up now. Soon my eyes took over my feet again and I was trudging again behind the steady silent stealth of Long-Life, who paused only long enough in places to find a new trail around thickets too tangled for the child he was leading.

It was almost pitch dark before we stopped, and we drank most of the water that was left, and ate some more pieces of the dried cheese. And then exhaustion won out over the effort of chewing and we simply laid down where we were and I fell off into a feverish sleep of unsettled dreams.

The following day we were up earlier; the sun was out bright and removed a little layer of my sadness. We had more pieces of cheese and then Long-Life took the lead again, this time choosing a path that led almost directly up the slope of a mountain. The early going was pleasant, on a winding trail through waist-high fern and flowers.

Some time after noon Long-Life stopped abruptly in his tracks, and lifted his nose to the air. I stopped too, and waited, and then a few seconds later I saw a movement in the trees ahead of us— up and to the left. And then out of the green stepped a family of brown deer with lovely white spots—first the father, a small buck with a little crown of antlers, and then a doe and, peeking around them, their fawn.

They caught sight of us instantly, and froze, and for the longest time between us all we just touched each other tentatively, with our eyes. Something inside me told me to offer them a *mandala:* this is a special prayer where we try to picture that the whole world, and every living thing in it, has already changed into a deathless paradise. And so I clasped my fingers before my heart in a special way and began to sing them the prayer, soft but clear as a bell. The father and the mother were startled, and stepped back into the shelter of the undergrowth. The fawn though slipped between them, and walked out unprotected onto the path before Long-Life and I, and stood entranced long after the final note of the song had died away into the trees.

And then we moved on, up to the right, and passed into vast sheets of brambles and thorns. I knew we must be working towards the peak of the mountain—Long-Life had his reasons, and I didn't question them. But from here on every step was a struggle, trying to force the cruel branches aside until I could slip by, or simply crawling under them with my belly digging into the moist earth.

Late in the afternoon I finally had to stop; I sat down, thought for a moment, and then hurried a few steps away and lifted my dress and had a violent case of diarrhea. I crawled back and laid down on the ground doubled up in cramps. Long-Life sat at my side quietly, looking down at me with doleful eyes. And I could see mixed with the mud caked on his once-fluffy tail a stain of yellow slime, and I knew he had been suffering too, from fever and the days of dried cheese. We drank then the last of the water, and he let me rest.

When I felt a little better Long-Life bent his head down and pushed against my hand, and raised his eyes ahead. Dusk was close, and we had to try to make the summit. I didn't question him at all; I just got up and pushed my way on. And then within thirty feet more we broke out of the brambles into empty sky, and a small flat stone ridge of mountaintop.

Long-Life walked immediately out to the far edge of the crest, and sat, gazing off to the southwest. I came up behind him, and caught my breath. There in the last weak glow of sunlight I could make out the dark green edge of the Western Forest, broken suddenly by The Rim: a slash of white granite shaped like a mighty V. And beyond that the sky was only a pale pink haze, covering the lowlands, and the canyon road to Katrin.

50.

The Slayer's Face

I woke up thirsty in a little clearing on the far side of the peak. My head was still a little dizzy from the fever, and I got a scare when I looked around and found Long-Life gone. I stood up with some difficulty and looked for him below in the trees, then turned around and spotted him through the brambles above: he was sitting still and attentive, gazing not ahead to the lowlands but back towards the forest we had come through, staring with the intensity of a hunter. And it occurred to me briefly that something else could very well be hunting us.

Then he was down in a flash brushing between my legs and forging ahead with what seemed like a quiet urgency. And I just picked up the baby sling and the empty water skin and followed, moving quickly. Neither one of us was ready for more of the dried cheese, although I knew time would change that.

We worked down off the mountain in a slight pale mist, and were back on level ground again by mid-morning. There at the bottom we sat for a few minutes; Long-Life seemed edgy, and kept turning his head to look back up the slope we'd descended.

We walked on only a few minutes more and then Long-Life stopped cold, his head held up and his ears cocked. I strained to hear what he heard and then it came to me—the buzzing sound of a swarm of bees. He angled off to the right towards the sound, and I followed—until we came to a strange tree that grew up a few feet and then split into three trunks.

There was a deep hollow in the middle fringed by a line of bees, drinking the rainwater trapped there. I got a branch from the ground and shooed them away as best I could, then picked up Long-Life and drank with him the brackish water until it was all gone. It made me think how quickly we get used to anything when the need is strong enough; and as we left I got a sting on the hand. It hardly hurt at all, but as we trudged on towards the Rim the poison began to work up my arm, mixing with the last of the fever to make me feel faint and troubled.

A few hours went by and we were skirting the edge of a meadow, following a deer trail around in a half circle close to the tree line. Long-Life it seemed was trying to make sure that we could never be caught out in the open, and this added a sense of foreboding to the dull headache I'd had since waking. There was a wind up from the lowlands, steady in our faces. Long-Life suddenly froze before me, with one front paw still up in the air, caught in half-step. The hair on the back of his neck bristled up, and about twenty feet ahead I saw a great grey wolf trotting down the path towards us.

He looked nearly six feet long, and stood as high as my waist. His head was down with the weight of a red mass of flesh and bone clutched in his jaws, and I knew the wind was blowing our scent the other way. He was almost upon us unknowingly when Long-Life and I both had the instinct to let him know we were there: I cleared my throat, and Long-Life gave out the most serious growl he could muster against such a beast.

The wolf's eyes shot up startled; he saw me first and simply dropped what he was carrying and flew off into the tall grass of the meadow, a long grey flash singing amidst the waves of brown, working through the wind. We watched after him in awe, and it brought on me all of a sudden the picture of Uncle, on the day that Grandmother fell, flashing crimson through the wheat behind the homestead. And then suddenly it really struck me that what was happening to us now might very well mean we would never see home again—never see Uncle or Father or Mother again—and a sharp pain came in my chest to make the thirst and fever seem all the more hopeless.

Long-Life glanced back at me over his shoulder, with sad eyes, and I knew he felt my thoughts. We stepped slowly ahead and came to the chunk of meat and broken bone in the middle of the path. I stopped, thinking that Long-Life might want to eat some of it; I didn't feel like I could. But he just sniffed at it and his hackles came up again, with a low eerie growl. He stepped around the flesh gingerly as if it were a snake, and I followed, and we pushed on towards The Rim, trying to leave the strangeness behind.

We broke out of the last of the Great Western forest just as the pink dusk began to settle again ahead of us. Suddenly we were on a long flat run of white granite, and we walked slowly to the edge of it, awed by the panorama laid out before us. It was the edge of our homeland, the vast wall of The Rim, which descended in a sheer cliff hundreds of feet to the lowlands. And these lands were still only an indistinct brown smudge below the haze of the sunset.

I realized then that we had come out a little too far north; we were up towards the middle of the side of the great V and would have to work back towards its point to find the way down the wall of The Rim.

We stopped and rested a few minutes more to admire the wall opposite us, fading from pink to a deeper crimson as the sun touched the horizon. And then I saw birds—dozens of huge black birds, nearly a hundred altogether. They were working upwards in a spiraling chimney over the blood-red cliffs—climbing on the updrafts bursting up the wall.

Long-Life stared up at them too, and then his eyes came down and he let out that growl again, the strange one. And I strained to see into the dusk and I could make out a huge dark figure making its way out onto that far cliff of blood. The shape was taller than a man, with massive humpbacked shoulders.

And it stood there still for a moment, and seemed to look across at the two of us, a tiny filthy little dog and a sick frightened girl. It twisted and pulled some ropes from its back, and then the naked body of a dead man fell from its shoulders to the cold rock of clifftop.

Suddenly I understood what we were seeing. It was the sky-burial; someone had died and according to the custom of the mountain people the flesh was being offered to the wild animals, to give some little sustenance back to the world that had fed the dead one for his or her whole life.

The dark man stepped back to coil his ropes back again. The great black ravens descended in a gabbling roar to tear at the flesh. They were pecking at the face and it dawned on me that it could have been Grandmother's dear face, or Tenzing's handsome features; that they might even have ended here, on this very rock. And I glanced at Long-Life's face turned towards the dark one silent as stone and I put my hand out to touch the fur on his neck for comfort but suddenly in the growing dark it was as if his skin were already gone, and it was only a grinning skull staring into the dark, and on my outstretched fingers too there were worms and maggots crawling already, eating what the birds and wolves had left nestled in the dirt.

And then an anger came over me and said *It will not be*, and I stood and walked slowly to the very edge of the cliff, so that the dark one, the Lord of Death, could see the face of the one who had come to slay him.

51.

The Singing Waters

Morning dawned bright and clear, and saw us at the mouth of the gorge that cut down The Rim to the lowlands. Here the pine-needle floor of the forest changed to wild granite and slate shattered like glass, with twisted oak for welcome shade. Within a half-hour's climb down the V we came upon a bright bubbling creek—I found a flat spot with a little pool and just jumped in dress and all. It was terribly cold and stole my breath away but I laughed for joy and let the water strip away the last of my sickness and fears. My brave little lion stood flustered on the bank but finally let me take him on my lap in a shallows, to wash the grime out of his lovely long hair. It felt then that we had truly escaped; that we were free of our old life, and its death. And somehow seeing Death himself—being reminded of why we had left, and why we were coming to Katrin—filled now the day and our hearts with sunshine, and a determination that would not be broken.

I sat in the sun dressed only in Uncle's white sage-cloth while my dress dried on a tree limb. Long-Life snuffled around and found a little cachet of acorns; I broke them up with stones, and picked out the shells, and then threw in the last of the wretched cheese and crushed it too. Then I mixed the two with some stream water in a bowl-shaped rock, and we ended up with a passable *sampa* paste. This is a gruel usually made with toasted barley flour, and enjoying a Tibetan's favorite breakfast made our spirits soar even higher.

The trip down the gorge, simply following the laughing stream, was a delight—with jays in the overhead announcing our arrival to the tiny gray squirrels caught drinking at pools. At two places the path beside the water gave way to high stone walls on each side; the creek-bed was a smooth water-worn rock that angled sharply down between them. At first I picked up Long-Life in my arms, stepped into the water, and cautiously tried to pick my way down. After a few falls I just tied my skirt up around my waist and slid down the rest of the way on my bottom, with Long-Life squirming bug-eyed in my arms But it was great fun, and medicine for the heart, and gave me a new appreciation for the soft sage's cloth.

By late afternoon we came suddenly out of the oaks into a kind of flat dusty plain that we call a *thang:* the long-awaited lowlands. The stream turned back here in a hairpin to the south, following the bottom of The Rim. But this was where Uncle had told the young sage to cut away across the flatlands, to the southwest. We stood still, the two of us, side by side at the edge of the cool murmuring water, looking out across that land. Dry, dead, rock and dust, broken only by a single miserable, stunted thorn tree.

Again it was the indomitable Long-Life who eventually stepped back, and went to the edge of the stream, and began to lap up all the water his belly could hold. He glanced up at me once and then I understood and came and drank all I could too. Then I filled Father's water skin as tight as it would go; and with the sun descending hot and bright we stepped ahead into the desolation, Long-Life's little paws raising tiny billows of copper dust with every resolute step.

52.

Power Unwanted

We walked straight on through sunset and kept moving: we both knew it would be easier going at night, for as long as we could keep it up. The moon rose early and had a bad feeling to it, darkened by the dust of the *thang*, even though I guessed it was only a day from full. That meant it was only a week since the magical last battle in the courtyard of the warriors; but that magic was far gone now.

I felt the sage's cloth ride my hips as we walked in a dull unbroken straight line; and I thought that although I was nothing of a sage the cloth almost made me feel the power of one at times. And it was one such time tonight, for I felt something coming that had not yet come; I could feel it pressing in from the hours ahead of us as surely as a hand pressing the dry land beneath our feet. And it was an evil hand.

Long-Life sensed it too but pulled himself bravely on to meet it. His tail was dragging flat now across the dry powder of the dirt—he was very tired, or very afraid, or both. But he kept on, and we walked naked across the naked flat land, bathed in moonlight and shadow.

53.

Far Enough to Lose the Way

The moon was nearly set, with dawn at its heels, before we were finally forced to stop. From sheer formality we laid down at the foot of a thorn tree that had nothing to shade us from the cruel sun to come. In a kind of panic I realized that the water-skin was already half empty; I could hardly recall us drinking at all.

Neither of us slept well; that dead land was surprisingly noisy when we fell still—rustles of slithering things and sudden bursts of feather-sounds just overhead. Long-Life seemed increasingly sad and tense, lifting his little head from my chest constantly to check the air, bristling even when he dozed off.

For want of anything else to do we rose only a little after the sun, eyelids dry and red from the dust and failed sleep. Again we trudged to the southwest, and I began to fear that we had lost our bearings during the night walk. I constantly scanned the way ahead but could see nothing but the dull red dust, stretching to some faint blue mountains low on the horizon—far further than we would ever be able to go.

A few hours later we were straggling on side by side, heads down tired, worrying about when to drink the last few gulps of water. Long-Life suddenly came up short, and luckily habit made me stop in the very same step. The red earth disappeared a few inches further, dropping several hundred feet into a wondrous canyon.

The first thing you saw was water—from up here at the top it was only a thin silver band drawn down the center of the canyon floor. In some places it spread out over huge flat banks, flowing only a few inches deep, bubbling over bright round sun-washed stones of every color. In other places it collected in blue crystal pools, hedged in on each side by wide green trees like sycamores.

Long-Life gave a tired bark of success, staring down excited at the water. I stepped back a few yards and looked again towards the canyon—from here it was almost completely invisible, the rust-colored sandstone of the opposite wall blending into the ground at my feet. I shook my head in wonder and we began to work south along the edge, looking for a way down.

We walked straight past the trailhead but further on we looked back and saw a comfortable path cutting down across the wall, worn flat by deer and wild sheep. We circled around and found the entrance, like a step into thin air. A quarter hour later I was sitting luxuriously in a crystal-clear pool, beneath an ancient overhanging oak, while Long-Life sat in the grass beneath it.

For a few minutes it seemed idyllic and then—as such things always go—doubts of a new kind began to assail me. The fact was that, from here, I had absolutely no idea which way to go to find Katrin. And freed from the thirst, I suddenly became aware that I was painfully hungry. Long-Life echoed my feelings; he stood up and began pacing nervously, looking first upstream, then down, unsure of himself really for the first time.

I decided on downstream, since I knew that all streams lead eventually to rivers that lead sooner or later to people. Within an hour the canyon opened into yet another canyon, with its own stream joining ours. I took off Grandmother's sweaty boots happily and carried Long-Life across to a larger deer path on the other side. We repeated this process several more times before it suddenly dawned on me that the canyon was really a confused maze of branch canyons, and that working back up the way we had come I would never be able to recognize which branch we'd started from. And then I just shrugged in my mind; there was no going back anyway, and the canyon was simply confirming the fact for us.

There were places where the path climbed up above the stream and ran across the cliff faces perilously; in one spot the way was torn out by a rockfall and I had to pick up Long-Life and jump across. It made me feel brave and independent; generally I find heights very frightening, but there was nothing else to do, and no one else to help.

In another place the path unfurled smoothly along the side of the water and then simply stopped before a huge boulder as high as my shoulders. Here I put Long-Life into the baby sling, flat against my back, and fought my way up on top of the rock. And then behind it was a whole field of boulders of almost exactly the same size and shape—as if some giants used the stones for marbles and kept them stuffed here in the pocket of the canyon between games.

Getting over stretches like this was more dangerous though than the jumps on the cliffs: there were spaces underneath where you could crawl between some of the boulders, but these little tunnels always ran into a dead end, or snake nests

I knew. And so finally I simply had to leap from one rounded top to another, knowing that if I slipped I would break a leg and die there, with no one to find me.

It was well into dusk when we came to another crossroads in the canyons, and forded across to a wide beach of pebbles. As soon as I set Long-Life down his nose came up and his ears flattened back, and he trotted off downstream without a moment's hesitation. I hurried after him, slipping over the round wet stones in the grayness, and we pushed our way through a tight thicket of reeds and thin young oaks.

And suddenly ahead there was a small fire; we froze for an instant and then Long-Life doubled back under my feet and dropped in the reeds—I scurried after him.

54.

Long-Life's Gift

I recalled Uncle's warning to the young sage that these canyons were used by highwaymen and bandits to travel with impunity north and south through our whole area of Tibet. On the other hand there was an exquisite aroma of dinner being fried in a skillet over the fire. I could see the same thoughts crossing Long-Life's face in the reflection of the firelight.

One moment his eyes were gazing off frightened to the side, calculating the chances of our getting past the fire without being spotted. I checked too, but it didn't look hopeful: just beyond the clearing there was a dark pool on this side of the stream, with a canyon wall ascending from the water in two huge pillars. Between the spires came the sound of a smaller spring falling into the pool from somewhere higher on the cliff face.

In the next moment Long-Life's eyes were back on the fire, and the food. In one way it didn't matter if we got past this spot undetected, since if we didn't have something to eat soon we couldn't go on much farther anyway. And so we decided to wait, and watch—perhaps the people would end up being a party of kind-hearted travelers. And if they were bandits, well perhaps later on they might sleep, and leave some scraps of dinner in reach.

There was a scuffling sound out across the other side of the fire; the bushes parted and a lone man stepped out of the dark into the red light. He was tall and gangly; across his shoulder was a rough, grimy nomad's cloak. Strapped to his belt was a long cruel knife; he pulled it out in a smooth, practiced motion and poked at something in the pan, which brought his head down close to the light.

His hair was covered in a shabby fur-skin cap, and he hardly seemed to have a forehead at all—this and the way he jabbed his blade dumbly over the fire gave him a frightening, almost witless look.

I considered just walking out and trying to trade him something—maybe my shawl—for some of the food, but something Father had always said came loud into my mind: "Try to make a deal with a stupid man and he will only hurt you." And this one was, and would.

"Gotcha!" and a huge strong hand is twisting the strap of the baby sling around my neck. And then I'm down on the ground and he's dragging me across the stones to the fire and Long-Life is choking and howling in fear with his neck in the other fist. And the skinny man is up in a flash with the knife out front and then his face lights up in a wicked grin.

The hand shoves me down at the fire but doesn't let go of the loop around my neck and I'm fighting for breath and the other hand simply throws Long-Life over the flames into the dark—he lands in a crumple. And I look up with a gasp at a wicked filthy smile and bulging bloodshot eyes and a nose that comes out and then down in a huge evil curving arc. He forces my head down to his mud-covered black boots and he pulls out his own knife, waving it in the air.

"Damn! Strangest things ya find just wanderin' around in the dark!" and the blade comes down in a swoop and taps me flat on the head and then flashes to the pan to spear a slice of sizzling meat. And he eats it with pig sounds and the grease is falling down hot on the side of my head.

The skinny one sits back down and leers. "Whatcha gonna do with her?"

"Dunno," says the big one, between bites. "If she's nice, maybe have us some fun, sorta for dessert. If she's not, suppose we just kill her, say?"

The knife comes down again and slashes open the side of the baby sling. The skinny one reaches over and shakes out Grandmother's shawl, and Father's waterskin, and throws them disgusted on the ground. "Yep, reckon that's all there is to do with her. Ain't nothin' worth nothin' here."

The big one just grunts and swallows—his hand on the loop tightens up steadily and my cheek now is in the dirt, and all I can see is the boot and the fire.

He chews—I can hear him chew—my ears are ringing and I'm afraid I'll pass out.

"Dog's back up," says the skinny one.

"Don't matter," grunts the big one. "Too scrawny to fry, too scared to bite." I hear his knife in the pan again, and the grease is falling on me. I can see Long-Life in the corner of my eye, at the edge of the fire.

"Long-Life," I choke. And then I say *"Om mani padme hum,"* the prayer that Long-Life used to do for table scraps.

And the big one says, "Ah, look at that. She's all scared and doin' prayers already."

But Long-Life understands and he's up on his two back legs in the firelight whining out his *"Om mani…"* and the skinny one says "Take a look at that will ya!" and then I scream out the *bam!* that Father taught him and from sheer reflex Long-Life launches his little body at the piece of meat suspended on the big one's knife. The skillet flies up and the skinny one is screaming with hot oil burning into his arm and the big one falls to the side and in an instant Long-Life and I are up and running in the dark down near the pool.

But the big one rolls fast like a cat and he's up again after us with a firestick brandished over his terrible face and suddenly we're back against a great boulder and I look out beyond and cry in fear—it's all boulders, only the huge boulders, for as far as I can see and I turn around and the big one is flying down upon me and suddenly Long-Life is out in between, like a tiny white flash across the ground. And he pauses once and looks back over shoulder with those beautiful brown eyes and the whites all showing in terror and I feel his fear and I see the gift he will give in spite of it and his eyes say once, "Run" and he turns back to face the big man.

And I cry out again "No!" but Long-Life leaps one last time and takes down the arm and the torch with his cruel tiny teeth. And the big one roars in pain and there are steps running behind him and there's a loud slapping sound and then nothing but silence and dark and the race of my own breath as I burrow down into the darkness, between the great stones, crawling for my life.

55.

The Point of No Choices

A rock stops me once and I have to turn right and then right and it's a dead end. I crouch in the dark amidst the boulders and try not to sob.

"Wicked cut ya got there."

The big one just grunts in anger.

"Well he won't never be bitin' nobody again, that's for sure," says the skinny one, and I strain my ears and the silence tells me that Long-Life is gone.

And then the torches are waving up above me and there is nothing but deadly silence broken by an occasional "Over there," or "Nothing." I know it is only time before they find me. And the only way to go is back towards them.

Almost to the clearing there was another opening among the boulders, off towards the cliff. And a few feet later my knees were in freezing water. The pool; another dead end.

And then a light came down close behind and in desperation I got down on my belly and pulled myself into the black water, until I was out free of the stones, crouching in the water, only my eyes and nose above the surface.

"Thought I saw something over here," and the other torch came close too. Sooner or later they would think to check the pool.

I looked to the canyon wall with the water cascading down: a flat sheer face. But off to the side there was one of the pillar-shapes, a chimney that came down out in front of the wall. It had cracks and ledges working across it up as far as I could see. And my fear of high places came on strong inside but behind it was a growing sense of fury—fury for the Lord of Death. And so stooping still I pushed silent into to the base of it and began to climb.

I didn't look down; I couldn't see anything up. At times I felt the torchlight on my back but I think they simply didn't think to look upwards. And I just found one crack at a time and pushed my fingers into it and pulled myself up another few inches. My legs were shaking from the cold and fear and I knew my dress was leaving a trail of water along the stone for the men to follow later. But I just climbed.

And then my hand went up searching for the next crack and the stone above was only flat. With joy I pulled myself up over that last ledge, to the top of canyon.

Except it was not the top of the canyon— only the top of the chimney rock, and that itself split here into two points. Each point had only just enough room to put one foot down, straddling empty space. And I crouched there and stared ahead into the darkness between the top of the chimney and the sheer wall of the canyon. It was too dangerous even to try looking down behind me, a drop of seventy or eighty feet to the boulders and the two men. In fear and cold and sadness then I just squatted there, perched in the air, knowing there was no way to go.

56.

Falling in Darkness

For the first time in my life I was literally frozen by my doubt. I simply crouched there on my haunches, too afraid to move. I could hear the men below still searching, and I could feel the anger of the big one growing with pain and frustration—growing into bloodthirst. And then I realized that my legs were falling asleep in the cold, and that when they did I would fall anyway.

Suddenly the full moon broke over the opposite rim of the canyon, back behind my left shoulder. It bathed me in a brilliant white light, and I knew then that the first man to look up would see me. But the moonlight also crept slowly down the wall of the cliff across from me, and it was then that I saw the path.

It was just a ledge really—not much more than a foot wide, cutting diagonally down the cliff.

One end stretched up into the dark to my left, and the other came down and stopped at the place where the spring water flew off the cliff, in a long waterfall to the pool.

From where I was at the top of the chimney, the ledge on the other side was about a fifteen foot drop. But the distance between the chimney and the cliff was impossible to judge.

And then I heard the voices of the men again behind me, and I thought of Grandmother and Tenzing lying dead out on one of the cliffs, and Long-Life's warm little body pressed against my chest at night, and now its warmth all leaked out, lying cold and bloody in the dirt below—and somehow then I saw all the people I had ever known, all the living creatures I had ever known, and those I had never known but who lived, warm and alive, and I felt the Lord of Death scrabbling for them, clawing at them, at their throats, and then he was the two men behind me and I decided, there, once and for all, that I would stand and fight him, fight for even the chance of learning how to kill *him*, once and for all, for all the warm life that exists in this and every world.

And so I looked across at the ledge, and I saw a stone coming up out of the cliff face that threw a shadow, a shadow that was just the shape of Uncle's face. And I took it as a sign and I turned around balancing on the two steps, and I bent down and jammed my shoulders into the space between them, and let myself down with my feet dangling in the air, as far as I could, my back to empty space. And when I could see Uncle's face over my shoulder I let go and pushed off and fell back into the dark.

57.

The Cave

I slammed into the cliff wall and it knocked the breath out of me but the ledge was right there, under my feet, and my feet held. Stones clattered down, and below the voices called excited to each other. I knew they would be up in a moment, if they could find a way.

The tiny ledge path to my left surely led to the canyon rim, and I knew too they would spot it easily and be waiting at the top if there was another way up. I looked a few feet to my right, to where the spring flowed off the rock, and then craned behind to see further up the little gorge it descended.

I put one foot in the water and kept one on the stone and boosted myself up an outcrop shaped like a giant step. Above that there was enough space to set both my feet on the rock, and I clambered up another step. This shelf widened out further, with a clump of straggly bushes to my left. Again I set my hands up on the next step, this one as high as my shoulders, and began to boost myself up.

And then against my face there was a little puff of air and a snapping sound, and a beam of moonlight struck a shape only inches in front of my face: the open hood of an emerald viper, poised, ready to strike.

I froze; I was too frightened to move, and I knew I would die if she only brushed me once. But the viper simply stood there, poised, like a sentry barring the way. A gentle hiss came out, like a sigh, as if to say simply "This is not the way." And suddenly it seemed right and I let myself back down slow, and crouched on the ledge.

Not down, not up, but not out here in the open either. I stepped over to the bushes to see if I could hide behind them.

And there in back was a little hole in the rock, not much wider than my hips. I crouched and reached in with one booted leg, to see if my lady viper might have a family there. But it was silent and finally the fear of the men pushed me on, and I crawled in. Everything was pitch black, except for the little circle of moonlight in the front.

I crawled back and suddenly realized the cave was tall enough to stand up in. It went on about fifteen feet and then the ceiling sloped down towards the floor, and in the very back there was a little pile of very old, hard wood. Someone had lived here.

And I sat down with a stick in my hand, determined to watch the soft circle of light throughout the rest of the night. I think it was only a few minutes though before the exhaustion and grief came down and pushed me into a fitful sleep—broken by half-dreams of a dark blanket of gentle, frightening spiders on long spindly legs, descending from the roof to cover me over.

58.

The Sun Rises in My Life

I woke at daybreak—soft light from the sun to come was filtering in through the hole. Suddenly I remembered the spiders, and looked up to see a trembling mass suspended from the stone overhead, just settling down to a day's sleep. I shivered and then heard the steps.

They were the soft shuffle of sandals—no ruffian jackboots, I knew—and they made a delightful rhythm as they came down the path below my ledge. And then they stopped I guessed at the spring, and I heard something heavy like a pot set down, and then a soft high humming that sounded like one of Uncle's lovely chants. I crept to the opening, kept my face low behind the bushes, and gazed down.

There was a tiny figure, its back to me, kneeling before the spring to fill a brown clay jar with the cold sparkling water. I would have thought it a child, but folded around the delicate frame were soft, faded maroon robes, stitched in the distinctive pattern reserved for elder monks.

He rose then gracefully and turned towards me to settle the jar inbetween his arm and hip—I pulled my face back instantly. And when I looked back he was fiddling with his monk's shawl, the way they always do, his arm out long over the cliffside waving a flap of the cloth. He turned the other way and paused for a moment, gazing down the length of the canyon, and then the little song of his steps retreated back up the path.

I hid there in the bushes for a few minutes to think, but I already knew what I would do. I felt a deep trust for this odd little monk already; his presence of those few moments hung still there in the very air, leaving some ineffable fragrance. Surely he would help me, or help me find help.

And so in the soft light before the dawn I let myself down to the path, and walked cautiously up towards the rim of the canyon. I hugged the wall to my right, trying to stay out of sight from below. Neither had I any wish to see Long-Life's dead body in the daylight.

The path came out on the rim, followed it for a short distance, and then angled off from the edge, which dropped several hundred feet sheer to the canyon floor. I came around a little point and stopped breathless.

I stood on a great crag of rock about a hundred yards across. It had a bit of a bowl shape that sloped down away from the edge of the canyon, with several tall pinnacles of stone scattered across the edges of the bowl. From there the ground fell off in a sharp slope to a wide green valley that spread west as far as I could see. To the south the stone points continued but lower, in a gentle string that followed the edge of the canyon and ended in some rounded brown mountains, several miles distant.

I walked to a short line of bushes at the side of the path and crouched down behind them, my back to the rim and the empty sky behind it. Down below, nestled in the bowl, was a little square house. It had a thatched roof and rough walls made of stacks of loose stone, with mud plaster daubed here and there.

Joined to one corner was another small square dwelling, and nestled out behind them was a very odd little garden, with rows of spring green spreading in a fan. At this I shook my head a bit; winter seemed to have left this little land long before the rest of the world.

Then behind me someone cleared their throat softly and I jumped in fright and looked back to the rim and suddenly the dawn sun breaks glorious golden over the canyon and standing in the center of it impossibly perched on the very edge of the precipice is that little old monk, his arms opened wide with the rays of sunlight bursting out behind them. And I still can't see his face for the brightness behind him but I hear his high squeaky voice ring out like a tiny crystal bell and it says, "Come, have some tea."

59.

The Story We Share

"Men," I stuttered, "danger," and he nodded slightly and said only "Gone." And he led me down into the soft humble warmth of the house—just a single room, really. He put me down on a threadbare little rug over the clean simple coolness of the stone floor, and busied himself in a corner in the back, at a simple hearth.

There was a tiny old wooden bed along the back wall, and above it a cheerful little window which let out to the bright green splash of the garden, and darker emerald of the valley below. To my left as I faced the window was a simple altar— more stones stacked atop each other, with several rough planks of wood and upon them the warmth of a few tenderly cared-for images of angels. Tiny fresh flowers were sprinkled among them, with little cups too of fresh spring water, and small finger-size pastries.

But most importantly, there above the bed— as in Uncle's yurt—hung a rough little wooden cabinet. One door was opened a crack to reveal neat little stacks of ancient holy books: loose sheets of parchment wrapped in worn, gaily-colored cottons and silks.

And then the little old monk leaned over me gently and pushed a bowl of piping-hot tea into my hands, and silently set another bowlful on a rickety little wooden table at the side of the bed. And then like all the Lamas he got up and sat down cross-legged on the bed—which served as his only chair during the day. He sang a quiet little prayer to offer the tea to all the Angels in the world, and then nodded for me to drink.

Whenever he took a sip I stole a glance at his face—it was worn and wrinkled everywhere with age; he had taut thin lips with ends chiseled sharply into corners at his cheeks: the lips of someone who had paid much hardship to learn the art of silence. Amidst the fine spider's web of wrinkles thrown across his eyes and forehead, grey-brown eyes burned young with fire and steel, belying the gentleness of his manner—soft wool over an iron anvil.

He stayed silent and sipped silent and let me steal my glances, until he was satisfied that my heart was settled.   The tea was a good strong Tibetan brew with fresh milk and salt and butter; it filled me full as any breakfast.   And then he said simply, "What shall I call you?"

"My name is Friday, Elder One," I replied.

I paused for a moment, and then asked him the same, with the special words of respect we use in our language: "And when I dare to speak your own name, Elder?"

And he answered then simply, "They call me... Katrin."

The very sound of the name threw my mind into a whirl.   And there are special ways, you see, traditions, that have been followed for centuries, for approaching a Master, and asking them to be your Teacher; and they require months of preparations and consideration and solemn pronouncements, but in that startled moment of confusion all I managed was "Katrin! Master Sage! I... Death! All dead, or... dying! So... I need to... I need, to know! To be... to do. The healing. Oh you *must* teach me!" And I threw myself forward on my knees, knocking the little wooden table over on its side.

The droopy eyelids came up sharply like tent-tops propped by a pole, and the steel eyes burned down into my face. But he said nothing, and I was afraid, and it suddenly struck me that this frail little creature didn't look anything at all like a Master Sage.

"You are… you are… Katrin; I mean, Katrin the Master Sage?" I asked stupidly.

He gave me a wry smile that quickly vanished. "Katrin I am; only Katrin, a tiny weak old monk, as you can surely see."

He stared down at the tea in his hands for another long moment, and then set the steel eyes on me again, studying my face intently. Then finally he said, "And the thing you ask… the thing you ask to learn, it is a very serious thing." He paused again, and his eyes fell silently, as if seeking words beneath the surface of the tea.

"And even if I knew—a little—about this… healing… well I could never teach it to you." A sharp flash of pain burst through my chest. He saw it.

"I mean, without knowing… without knowing exactly who you are, and why you want to learn this thing; why you, why someone so young, why just a girl." These last words stung me and he paused once more, studying his bowl, turning it in his fingers. And then suddenly he looked up again, his eyes twinkling.

"And how you found me! How you found this hermitage! I don't believe *anyone* has ever reached this place the way you did!" He leaned over into my eyes and my life again and he said, "So now tell me child, from the beginning, and leave nothing out."

And so I told him, everything, everything you have read here. And I know it may seem long to you and I am no eloquent writer. I know too that you live in another world and another time altogether, in great cities that we could never have even imagined, with incredible machines to serve your needs that would have seemed pure magic to us.

But I also know that living within those mighty buildings, surrounded by your unthinkable inventions, you too are dying. And I know that my own story is not special, because I know that you too have a Grandmother, and that she is dead, or nearly so. I know that if you have a brother like Tenzing that you have lost him too, or will. I know that you may keep a small dear friend like Long-Life, and you and I both know that he or she will leave you too, or you will leave them.

And so my story is nothing special, I know. But that is exactly why I have told it to you, and why I told it to my Master, Katrin. Because now the story changes—and the story of every life ever lived on this planet can change as well. Because death and sickness and growing old you see are not something that has to happen to anybody. That is an old evil idea, and it is a very wrong idea.

These things have only happened up to now only because people did not know the healing—the healing which I give to you here now, as Katrin gave it to me.

*Watch for the exciting conclusion
of Katrin appearing soon
in Volume Two!*

About the author

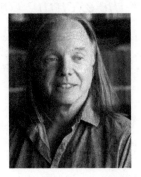

Geshe Michael Roach was born in Los Angeles in 1952, and grew up in Phoenix, Arizona. In 1975 he graduated with honors from the Religion Department of Princeton University, and is also a recipient of the McConnell Scholarship Prize from the University's School of Public & International Affairs. He has as well received the Presidential Scholar Medallion from the President of the United States at the White House.

Michael is the first westerner in the 600-year history of Tibet's Sera Mey Monastery, one of the largest in the world, to be awarded the degree of *Geshe* (Master of Buddhism), after completing the required 25-year course and public examinations. In 1987, he founded the Asian Classics Input Project, which trains and pays refugees to digitalize the classic books of the East, and provides thousands of ancient manuscripts online without charge.

The ACIP project led to the discovery and preservation of several dozen ancient texts of yoga, and in 2003 Michael founded the Yoga Studies Institute to translate, distribute, and teach these authentic, ancient systems of yoga exercise. His novel about a young woman who discovers and shares the deeper teachings of yoga, *How Yoga Works*, is a bestselling classic found in many languages, in yoga studios around the world.

By the same author

How Yoga Works:
*Healing Yourself and Others with
the Yoga Sutra*

The Garden: *A Parable*

The Diamond Cutter:
*The Buddha on Strategies
For Managing Your Business &
Your Life*

The Karma of Love:
*100 Answers for Your Relationship,
From the Ancient Wisdom of Tibet*

The Essential Yoga Sutra:
Ancient Wisdom for Your Yoga

King of the Dharma:
The Illustrated Life of Je Tsongkapa

Karmic Management:
*What Goes Around Comes Around,
In Your Business & Your Life*

The Eastern Path to Heaven:
*A Guide to Happiness
From the Teachings of Jesus
in Tibet*

The Tibetan Book of Yoga

Asian Classics Institute:
❖ The 18 Books of the
Foundation Course In Buddhism
❖ The 10 Buddhist Meditation
and Practice Modules
❖ The 18 Books of the Diamond-
Way Course In Buddhism

Door to the Diamond Way

Three Treasures:
A Buddhist prayer book

China Love You:
The Death of Global Competition

The Principal Teachings of
Buddhism

Emptiness Meditations:
*Learning How to See
That Nothing Is Itself*

The Golden Key:
*Difficult Questions
In the Mind-Only School of
Buddhism*

The Prayers of the Seven
Buddhas: *The Longer Sutra of the
Medicine Buddha*

All the Kinds of Karma:
*The Correlations Between
Our Actions & Their
Consequences,
According to the Buddha*

A Door to Emptiness:
*The Crucial Teaching
For Touching the Diamond World*

Sunlight on Suchness:
The Meaning of the Heart Sutra

Sunlight on the Path to Freedom:
*A Commentary to
The Diamond Cutter Sutra*